T0155217

A Place in the Country

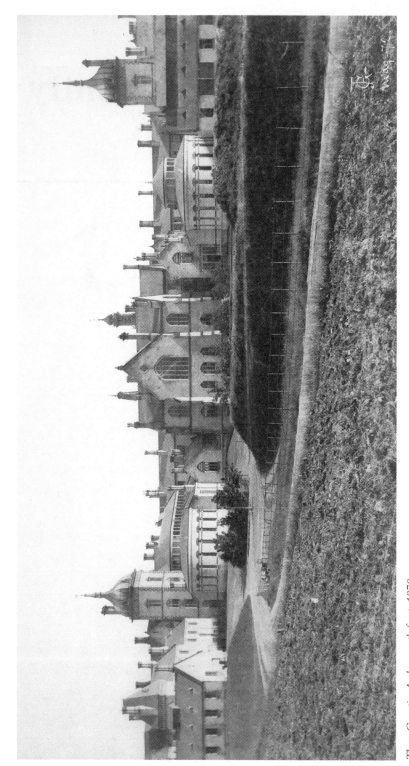

Three Counties Asylum north front, 1870

A Place in the Country

Three Counties Asylum
1860–1999

Judith Pettigrew,
Rory W. Reynolds
& Sandra Rouse

Hertfordshire Publications
an imprint of
UNIVERSITY OF HERTFORDSHIRE PRESS

First published in Great Britain in 2017 by
Hertfordshire Publications
an imprint of
University of Hertfordshire Press
College Lane
Hatfield
Hertfordshire
AL10 9AB

A longer version of this book was published in 1998 by
South Bedfordshire Community Health Care Trust.

British Library Cataloguing in Publication Data
A catalogue record for this book is available from the British Library

ISBN 978-1-909291-50-8

Design by Arthouse Publishing Solutions Ltd
Printed in Great Britain by Hobbs the Printers Ltd

Contents

Acknowledgements

Our particular thanks go to Maria Gamble, who was the team administrator of the Secure Services at Fairfield Hospital at the time we wrote the first edition of this book, and to the then members of Fairfield's Occupational Therapy Department who were unstinting in their support throughout the project. A number of people kindly read early drafts of the original manuscript. For their insightful comments and criticisms, we are indebted to Michael Rouse, Dot Slater, Louise Weber, Steve Iwasyk and Irene Howard. We are very grateful to the staff at the Bedfordshire and Luton Archives and Records Service and especially James Collett-White for sharing with us his expert knowledge of the Fairfield Hospital Archive. Our thanks also go to Anna Lorenzetto, Edna Gooderson, Evelyn Brown, Jackie Morris, Rose De Roeck and Ann Thomas for their generous secretarial support and assistance.

The authors would like to single out Nicholas Bridges for his expertise on architectural history and advice on specialist sources. We are very grateful to Stuart Elliott for technical advice. Other people who helped out in numerous ways are Jean Griffin, Richard Waterhouse, Claire Burton, Owen Davis and Caroline Edwards.

Illustrations

Introduction

For almost a century and a half, the care of the mentally ill in Bedfordshire, Hertfordshire and Huntingdonshire was provided by the Three Counties Asylum (TCA). As the era of institutional care of the mentally ill came to a close, Fairfield Hospital, as it came to be known, closed its doors in 1999. When it had opened as the Three Counties Asylum in 1860, asylum care was considered to be an important new approach to the treatment of the mentally ill. Under the terms of the 1845 Lunacy Act, the mentally ill were to be provided with humane treatment in specialised and carefully monitored institutions which were to replace the harsh treatment meted out to them in private madhouses, prisons or workhouses.

Despite the intentions of the lunacy reformers to create therapeutic environments, the large overcrowded county asylums did not achieve their promise. Little medical or psychiatric treatment was available until the mid-twentieth century, and while the excesses of the earlier era of private institutions were much less evident, aspects of life in the large asylums were harsh and often dehumanising. This was an era that was marked by both care and coercion. New drug treatments in the post-war period, combined with the growing awareness of the problems of long-term institutionalisation, heralded a return to community care. Several discussions of this dramatic change in therapeutic regimes have appeared in academic writings on the history of psychiatry, for example, Jones, Scull, Shorter and Porter.[1] It is a story which has also been told in the context of individual hospitals, such as Cashman's history of the Bedford Asylum, Clark's partly autobiographical account of Fulbourn Hospital, Cambridge, Valentine's work on the Horton Hospital, Epsom, Russell's account of the Bethlem Hospital and Crammer's history of the Buckinghamshire County Asylum.[2]

One of the problems with archival history is that the surviving data is predominantly that recorded by official bodies in compliance with regulatory agencies. Glimpses of day-to-day life in the early asylum are rare. Thus, the view of asylum life for the first hundred years is primarily what can be culled from official records such as those of the Visitors' Committee for the Commissioners in Lunacy, as recorded in monthly minutes and annual reports. This is a view of asylum management from the perspective of those whose connection with the institution was very tenuous. Reports of the asylum chaplain and the medical superintendent were subject to the scrutiny of the Visitors' Committee and the Commissioners in Lunacy, and were necessarily composed with that audience in mind.

The rhetoric of these documents and of Victorian psychiatry in general can seem lurid and demeaning by twenty-first-century standards. However, in the interests of historical accuracy, we make no attempt to censor our account but rather use whatever terms are appropriate to the era. Terms such as 'lunacy', 'idiocy' and 'imbecility' were the common currency of official mental-health records and legislation well into the twentieth century. The mentally ill have been variously labelled as 'inmates', then 'patients' and in the 1980s, as they moved out into the community, they became 'clients'. More recent terms include 'service users', or 'survivors'. Classification and the nomenclature of mental illness have altered substantially since the 1860s, as have the supposed causes and forms of insanity. The term 'schizophrenia', for example, was not coined until 1908 by the Zürich psychiatry professor, Eugen Bleuler. Bleuler was a follower of the German psychiatrist, Emil Kraepelin, who had labelled the condition 'dementia praecox' in the late nineteenth century. In the same era, the Commissioners in Lunacy set out a schedule of types of insanity (mania, melancholia, epilepsy, etc; see Appendix, p. 115) which restricted the possible forms to fourteen. All patients on admission to asylums had to be assigned to one of these categories. This label remained with the individual for the rest of their time in hospital – often a lifetime.

Record-keeping of accounts and ledgers involving any kind of expense or income was diligently carried out, including the costs of caring for patients and retaining staff. Yet the experiences of patients and staff are not chronicled. Until well into the twentieth century, case notes consisted of little more than a line or two a year indicating the patient's general state, often a whole year being recorded simply as 'no change'. All patient records were written in large general ledgers until 1912, when individual case files were instituted. Quarterly notes on patients were a requirement from the 1890s, though few, if any, were kept that systematically. It remained the norm for case notes of patients spending forty or fifty years in the hospital to consist of no more than two or three pages.

Despite the commonly held view that admission to a Victorian asylum was a life sentence, TCA, like other asylums, discharged significant numbers of patients. Patients, their relatives or the medical superintendent could request discharge. The requests were placed

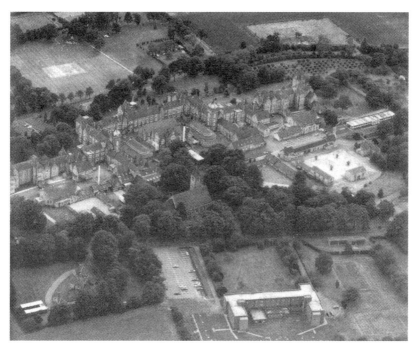

Figure 0.1 Aerial view of hospital and grounds

before the Committee of Visitors at their monthly meetings. The patients were usually seen in person by the Committee, who would decide on the basis of their presentation, in addition to the doctor's recommendation, if they were fit to be discharged. There was also an intermediary status of being allowed 'out on trial'. This meant that the patient was released into the responsibility of a relative or friend for a stated period of time. If things were going well, this time could be extended and ultimately could lead to full discharge.

Important, too, was the inter-relationship of the hospital and the local community. As a very large institution, having up to 1250 patients and several hundred staff, situated between the villages of Arlesey and Stotfold, the hospital both dominated and was intimately embedded in local community life. Four or five generations of families worked at the hospital. In the early years, the character of the hospital community was defined by the people of these villages who provided most of the staff. In the post-war era the villages themselves were redefined by the hospital as staff were recruited from overseas, and married and settled in surrounding communities.

Two histories of the hospital have been helpful in putting together the book. The resident chaplain, the Rev. Arthur Monk, wrote a pamphlet history to celebrate the hospital's centenary in 1960, and

Margery Burden's 1968 thesis chronicled the same era, providing valuable analytical material. The main historical source for TCA is the Fairfield Hospital Archive, deposited in the Bedfordshire and Luton Archives and Records Service. The collection dates from the initial plans for the hospital in 1852 through to its closure in 1999, and contains all official records, including reports, minutes, ledgers, case files, registers, drawings, photographs and correspondence. Other sources consulted include Quarter Sessions, census records, parish registers and local and national newspapers.

In this new edition of the book the text has been thoroughly checked so that any small errors that may have found their way into the original book will, we hope, have been corrected in this version. We have made some cuts too. The original book was in two parts – the first devoted to the history of the asylum and this is essentially what we present in this edition. The second part of the 1998 book was an oral-history section: a snapshot, if you like, of the remembrances and day-to-day experiences of identified staff and patients who were part of the hospital in its final days. However, many years have elapsed and, bearing in mind the right to personal privacy, we are unwilling to reprint these personal stories without each person's express consent. Sadly, it has not been possible to undertake the considerable research that this would entail and so we have, with some regret, chosen not to include the second part of the original book in this version.

Finally, our very grateful thanks to Jane Housham from University of Hertfordshire Press for inviting and encouraging us to re-visit *A Place in the Country* and work with her in making this second edition a reality.

Notes

1   K. Jones, *Asylums and After: A Revised History of the Mental Health Services*, Athlone Press, 1993; A. Scull (ed.) *Madhouses, Mad-Doctors and Madmen: The Social History of Psychiatry in the Victorian Era*, Athlone Press, 1981; E. Shorter, *A History of Psychiatry: From the Era of the Asylum to the Age of Prozac*, John Wiley & Sons, 1997; R. Porter, *A Social History of Madness: The World through the Eyes of the Insane*, Obelisk, 1989.

2   B. Cashman, *A Proper House: Bedford Lunatic Asylum 1812–1860*, North Bedfordshire Health Authority, 1992; D. Clark, *The Story of a Mental Hospital: Fulbourn 1858–1983*, Process Press, 1996; J Crammer, *Asylum History: Buckinghamshire County Pauper Lunatic Asylum-St. John's*, Gaskell, 1990; D. Russell, *Scenes from Bedlam*, Ballière Tindall, 1996; R. Valentine, *Asylum, Hospital, Haven: A History of Horton Hospital*, Riverside Mental Health Trust, 1996.

CHAPTER ONE

Planning and Building the Asylum

In 1837, the counties of Hertfordshire and Huntingdonshire began sending their 'pauper lunatics' to the Bedford Asylum. Built in 1812 by the Borough of Bedford for forty patients, it was not only running out of room for the living but also for the dead, since the burial ground of the nearby St Mary's Church was overflowing. By December 1839 there were 118 patients in the asylum and, despite all efforts to reduce the population, by 1843 it had grown to 136. In the winter of 1852, the visiting magistrates responsible for supervising the work of the asylum commissioned a survey with recommendations for improvements from Samuel Hill, the superintendent of the North and East Ridings of Yorkshire Asylum. The Yorkshire Asylum they considered 'a perfect model of a curative lunatic asylum, and Mr. Hill himself a most judicious exponent of all the requirements which an institution of the kind demands'.[1]

Hill was accompanied south by George Fowler Jones, a York architect. Together they inspected the asylum and forwarded their report to the Committee.

Hill's recommendations stressed the importance of what came to be called 'moral treatment' as developed by William Tuke at the York Retreat from 1796. Moral treatment called for a therapeutic environment of congenial surroundings, good food, fresh air and a routine of work, leisure and exercise. From this perspective, Hill concluded that the Bedford Asylum was no longer a suitable place of treatment for the mentally ill. While some patients were accommodated on the upper floor in dormitories, others had to sleep in the day rooms downstairs and even, he suspected, in the airing courts outside. Both wings of the asylum had such low ceilings that good ventilation was impracticable and in some rooms there were no fireplaces. The asylum was meant to be warmed by a hot-water apparatus but on the occasion of Hill and Jones's visit, some of the furnaces were under water because the natural springs underneath the building were unusually full.

Hill proposed improvements and alterations and added, 'in order to govern with mercy you must construct with judgement – you should aim to have no dark corners, obscure recesses closed with doors, or

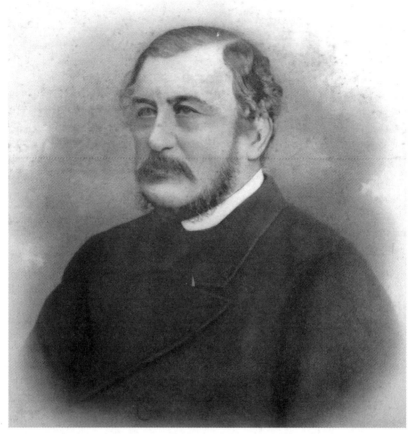

Figure 1.1 Marlborough Pryor, Chairman of the Visiting Committee, c.1860

blockaded windows'.[2] He went on to say that patients should be able
to look over the current 'dead walls' of the Bedford Asylum into light
and airy surroundings. It was clear that adapting a building originally
intended for 40 inmates to accommodate something in the region of
140 would be difficult. In the event, Jones's plans for extensions to the
Bedford Asylum proved too costly and the Court of Quarter Sessions
appointed a special committee with Thomas Charles Higgins as chair
to draw up proposals for the purchase of the land and the erection of a
new asylum.[3] The committee included Marlborough Pryor JP (1807–
69) from Weston Park near Baldock, who represented Hertfordshire,
and William Williams, the Mayor of Bedford.

The committee's first planning meeting had to be postponed
because a new application had been submitted. Cambridgeshire wanted
to join the original three counties of Hertfordshire, Bedfordshire and
Huntingdonshire to build an asylum for all four counties to use, the

cost to be shared between them. The initial approach had been made in a letter from the Clerk of the Committee of Visitors for the Union of Cambridgeshire, the Isle of Ely, and the Borough of Cambridge. A delegation from Cambridge put their case at the meeting in February 1853 and, as a result, it was agreed to recommend that a new asylum be built for the joint use of all four counties. Some 200 acres of land were to be purchased 'as near as may be to the Great Northern Railway'. The total cost for land and buildings was estimated at £70,000 and the counties of Hertford, Cambridge and Huntingdon were invited to unite with Bedford 'for the purpose of its construction'.

By the summer of 1853, David King, the Clerk to the Cambridge Visitors, wrote to say that his committee was impatient to hear something conclusive with regard to the plans being made. He proposed that 'the matter should be settled once and for all otherwise I fear the chance of our County uniting with the others will be at an end.' The Bedford contingent were principally responsible for the slow pace of development as they had reservations about moving the busy asylum out of town and were asking for compensation for the loss of income that would ensue. Theed Pearse, the town clerk of Bedford Borough, wrote in August to request the appointment of an independent arbitrator to settle the matter. It was at this point that the Cambridge Union refused categorically to give in to the demands of Bedford, and the Committee of Visitors of Cambridgeshire narrowly voted against the proposed Four Counties Asylum. This left the other three to proceed with plans for the new asylum which they proposed should be a building for about 500 patients called the 'Three Counties Asylum'.[4]

Selecting the Site

With Cambridgeshire removing itself from the planning process, the three counties of Hertfordshire, Bedfordshire and Huntingdonshire set about looking for a new site for their asylum. They initially set up a Committee of Visitors under the chairmanship of Marlborough Pryor. Samuel Wing was Clerk to the Committee. Bedfordshire had four representatives, including William Whitbread. Hertfordshire's four members included Pryor and the Marquis of Salisbury (who did not attend meetings). The Huntingdonshire contingent included James Rust, MP. Samuel Hill, the medical superintendent from York, had originally advised the Cambridgeshire Union about their plans for a new asylum on the outskirts of town at Fulbourn. He brought with him the York architect, George Fowler Jones, who had previously concentrated on designing and building churches, although he had worked with Hill on extending the York Asylum. Jones set about

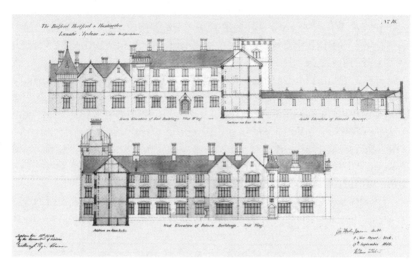

Figure 1.2 George Fowler Jones' plan of 1856 for the lunatic asylum at Arlesey

designing the Cambridge asylum and, in many respects, the Three Counties Asylum was built on a similar plan.

In January 1856, Jones was appointed architect for the new Three Counties Asylum.[5] This is the official version noted in the minutes. However, there is some evidence to suggest that he had been appointed earlier, or at least been asked to provide sample drawings, as there are plans for the new asylum under his name dated as early as 1853. In fact he had designs for an asylum for 500 patients ready to show the committee within three weeks of his official appointment.

The committee had already selected two sites that they thought might be suitable – Cadwell Farm in Ickleford near Hitchin owned by the Delmé-Radcliffe family and Arlesey Rectory Farm. Hill was invited to inspect and give his opinion about the suitability of the sites. He reported to the next meeting of the committee on 21 February that he could not approve of the Arlesey Rectory Farm site because of the 'heavy tenacious character of the soil which is altogether unsuited to the purpose of a lunatic asylum'.[6] On the other hand, he thought the Cadwell farm site offered distinct possibilities. It had a light workable soil (bearing in mind the land would have to be used for farming), an ample supply of water (essential in the days before piped water), a beautiful surrounding prospect, and close proximity to the main Great Northern Railway line between London and Edinburgh, which also connected to Bedford via the Midland Railway link.

However, doubts were expressed about the suitability of Cadwell Farm since there was no naturally flat area on the 170 acres to place a large asylum, the land being rather undulating. It was then suggested that land belonging to Major Wilkinson of Stotfold be inspected. Hill gave the 200-acre site a cursory examination and found the soil to be 'generally light and good', with gentle slopes and 'plenty of space on which to build an asylum with a SSE prospect'.[7] The plans to build on the Cadwell Farm site were, in any case, squashed by the Commissioners in Lunacy who felt that the uneven nature of land would create problems when supervising patients working outside. This appears to have caused some distress to Marlborough Pryor, who had spent time and money investigating the Cadwell option and was, without doubt, its main supporter.

At the 10 March meeting, it was decided instead to buy Major R. Hindley Wilkinson's 200 acres for £11,000. The Committee next sought to purchase another 50 acres to connect this parcel of land with the Great North Railway (GNR), which was about three quarters of a mile away.[8] This corridor of land was to become the Arlesey drive and tramway. At the same meeting, the resident engineer of the GNR, Benjamin Burleigh, showed his plans for making a tramway and footpath which would connect the asylum land with the village of Arlesey. The rail link would meet the GNR line near to Arlesey cement works and would run for about a mile across Arlesey's Hitchin Road and up to the new asylum. He estimated the cost of the road and tramway at £1,808 3s 4d for materials and labour, with a reduction of £628 16s if gravel should be found on the site (otherwise they would have to buy gravel). Burleigh pointed out that the consent of Arlesey Parish Council would also be needed for the line to cross the main street. Surprisingly, there is little mention of test borings for water. This oversight ultimately led to severe water-supply problems over the years, holding up some very necessary expansion.

After purchasing the 200 acres, the Committee had some difficulty buying the additional land for the tramway and road access. Earle Welby, who owned the land that the committee originally wanted, either did not want to sell or was hoping for a handsome profit by offering to sell at £200 per acre. This was at a time when local land was generally selling for £65 to £75 per acre. The committee refused the offer and turned their attention to a neighbouring field owned by Jonah King who agreed to a price of £65 per acre. The committee were able to buy the whole parcel of 57 acres for £2892.[9]

All contracts for land purchase had to await ratification by the Commissioners in Lunacy, who insisted on visiting the proposed site to ensure that it met with their specifications. Agreement was finally given in a letter dated 25 April 1856. The purchase of Wilkinson's and King's land went ahead in June of that year, and the site was readied for work to begin. However, it was to be three years and nine months before the first patients from Bedford asylum could be moved across to the new hospital and a great deal remained to be done to make the new asylum a reality.

Site Preparation and Building Works

The building of the tramway was a necessary part of the pre-construction phase as it would be used to bring all materials from either the brickworks in Arlesey (although not all the bricks used to construct the original main building came from there), or from other sources to the site. The GNR specified that they did not want the new tramway to connect to their main line and also revised the costs of laying the track upwards from £1808 3s 4d to £1995 7s 4d – a figure which was immediately accepted by the Committee. In order to make connection with the GNR, the Committee had no option but to purchase the freehold of an existing siding belonging to the Arlesey Cement Co for £650.

Burleigh, the GNR's resident engineer, was hired to oversee the construction. Jones estimated that about 30,000 tons of material would be required for the buildings and thus the tramway would save the Committee 9d per ton compared to the cost of transporting it all by road, giving a total saving of about £1000. The construction of the tramway included the building of a new station some one and a quarter miles south of the existing Arlesey station. The GNR agreed to stop two passenger trains in each direction there daily.

Burleigh's new rail link was to be a single-track standard gauge (4ft 8½in). Construction started 200 yards south of the proposed station, turning east through a 90° turn past the Lamb Inn (later the Admiral), almost immediately crossing what is now Hospital Road and intersecting Hitchin Road in Arlesey at the south end of the village. The GNR leased a parcel of land near the Lamb Inn to the Committee, which allowed the small road to be diverted for 20/- per year.

Burleigh quickly set to work and purchased rails from the Ebbw Vale Co., the biggest producer of railway lines in the country, for £624 2s 6d. His plans for the construction of the tramway and road were accepted by the Committee on 28 July 1856.[10] The scheme was to be undertaken by Charles Culshaw and included laying the track, with a road 18 feet wide alongside, plus hedging and fencing to afford protection. A 200-foot passing loop for the tramway was necessary just inside the asylum gates. The track then ran straight for about a quarter of a mile on the south side of what later became Arlesey Drive. As it entered the main site, it crossed the asylum approach road and entered a tightly curved cutting on a rising gradient for about another quarter of a mile.[11] There was a final 130-foot section of straight track which

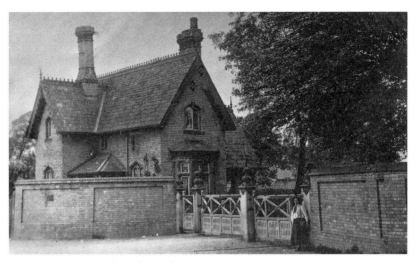

Figure 1.3 Entrance to the asylum, Arlesey Gate, c.1900

led directly to the site of the proposed new asylum. The soil from the cutting was banked on the north perimeter of the loop so as to provide a windbreak and was planted with trees for protection from the cold northerly winds.

The price of the tramway construction was £3164. The plantation along the line and at the northern edge of the site, including the raised earthworks, came to £1169. A further £810 was paid to the Arlesey Cement Co. for their weighbridge and weighhouse near to the Lamb Inn in Arlesey.[12]

One unusual feature of the plans was Jones's design for the terminus of the tramway to be within the asylum building. The Commissioners did not veto this proposal, but felt bound to comment on it: 'it is very unusual and extraordinary (not to say very unnecessary provision) to have a rail road under the very structure of the building at its terminus.'[13] They also requested that Burleigh add a short spur line to the completed track before it entered the cutting at the site of the proposed gas house, so that coal could be delivered. This was immediately done and by June 1857 Burleigh was able to report to the new Building Committee that all the necessary track had been laid, the station on the main GNR line erected and screening shrubs and fences had been put in place along the route of the tramway and road that formed the drive. The construction of the first buildings could now proceed.

On 9 March 1857, the minutes record that tenders had been received from eleven builders. The only local firm to bid, Jeeves of Hitchin, put in a tender for £73,786 but this was by far the most expensive estimate and the contract was awarded to William Webster of Boston, Lincolnshire. Webster had worked with Hill and Jones on the construction of Fulbourn Asylum and had been recommended by them. His tender came in at £53,626 and was the second lowest the committee received. The Committee awarded the contract to Webster, subject to agreement by the Commissioners in Lunacy, and the necessary funds being made available by the Courts of Quarter Sessions of the three counties.

Webster started work on 1 May 1857 by setting up his sheds and workshops along the east side of the Stotfold Road. A Building Committee had been inaugurated under the chairmanship of Marlborough Pryor to oversee and co-ordinate the efforts of the different contractors then working on the site. Pryor turned the first sod in a short ceremony and Webster was given permission to start work.[14] He began to sink the foundations of the asylum at once and found that, due to the high gravel content of the soil, it was necessary to excavate two feet further than Jones had planned in order to make the footings substantial.[15] Webster also dug the surrounding fields for gravel, sand and lime, and built the foundations from local Arlesey bricks.

With the building work substantially under way, the Committee of Visitors turned to the problem of providing sufficient water for the new asylum. They had bought the land on the understanding that a good well could be sunk without too much trouble and, in consequence, had only made one or two cursory borings before signing the purchase contracts. They estimated that about 10,000 gallons a day would be needed to satisfy the demands of the new building, but the subsequent bores were producing far less than this. It was a worrying situation and the Visitors' Committee reports include repeated warnings that if action was not taken, the building might be prevented from opening.

In July 1857, the Rev. James Clutterbuck of Long Wittenham near Abingdon in Oxfordshire was called in to see what could be done to increase the flow. Clutterbuck was a keen amateur geologist who had had some success with solving water shortage problems. He wrote the committee a long report detailing the problems and suggested that they drive into the main well shaft with horizontal cuttings to provide extra well heads, at the same time increasing the depth of the shaft to 73 feet. By the time of the opening of the asylum, the main shaft was some 6 feet in diameter and there were new headings ranged around for an area of 50 feet. Clutterbuck's proposals had worked well enough to allow the asylum to open and pump sufficient water for its needs.[16] As we shall see, though, accessing potable water was to remain an issue for the Three Counties Asylum and, indeed, would prove something of a nightmare when they sought to extend the institution some 13 years later.

Asylum Design

Before the nineteenth century, the mentally ill were housed in private madhouses or subscription hospitals where the predominant model was one of mechanical and physical restraint, usually accompanied by neglect and general ill treatment. This model underwent a dramatic change in the wake of the opening of the York Retreat in 1796. In 1791 a member of the Society of Friends had died in suspicious circumstances at the York Lunatic Asylum (founded 1777). The Society, angered by the asylum's refusal to allow visitors and disturbed by the death of one of their members, founded a new institution that was to be neither a hospital nor a madhouse but a 'retreat' for a small number of patients who could afford to pay for their upkeep. Largely conceived by William Tuke, the basis of care was something that came to be called 'moral treatment', under which he specified a regime of good food, fresh air, exercise and occupation in a congenial setting.[17]

After the turn of the century and with the rise of the social-reform movement, the County Asylums Act 1808 was passed. It included a provision for setting up county asylums with buildings to be paid for by the counties and patient rates paid by the parishes. The publication of *Description of the Retreat near York* by William Tuke's grandson Samuel Tuke in 1813 coincided with scandals of patient abuse at the York Lunatic Asylum and at the Bethlem Hospital (known colloquially as 'Bedlam') in London, and this raised the question of the monitoring of patient welfare. The subsequent County Asylums Act, passed in 1828, required regular inspection of all asylums by a committee of visitors appointed by the Secretary of State and the keeping of proper records.[18]

When the 1828 Act was passed, there were only nine county asylums, including the Bedford Asylum which had been built in 1812.[19] Between 1828 and 1842, another eight were erected. By 1839, the Middlesex Asylum at Hanwell was the largest in England with 1000 beds. In that year, John Conolly was appointed its Resident Physician. Conolly had written his MD thesis on insanity at Edinburgh in 1821 and published his *Inquiry Concerning the Indications of Insanity* in 1830. In the course of his research he had visited the Lincoln Asylum which had adopted the York Retreat's regime of moral treatment, emphasising a policy of non-restraint. Conolly immediately applied the model to Hanwell and demonstrated that it could be made to work in a large institution.

The controversies in the first half of the nineteenth century had led to demands for a body to be set up to oversee the provision of care for 'idiots, lunatics, imbeciles and epileptics'. Under the Lunatics Act of 1845, the Commissioners in Lunacy were made responsible for monitoring the management of all asylums, private madhouses and hospitals for the insane.[20] They were mandated to inspect all asylums once a year, and to deliver annual reports to the Lord Chancellor as to the condition of the asylums and the patients who were kept there. New regulations for the certification of insanity were instituted, and detailed records of admissions, deaths, discharges, forms of restraint, medical treatments and so on were required, as well as the keeping of visitors' books and regular reports by the medical officers of the asylum.

These regulations heralded an era of officialdom and brought into the public sphere the need for sufficient humane institutions to house the growing number of mentally ill. The watchdog role of the Lunacy Commission reduced the overt abuses of the old system and placed a new emphasis not on medical treatment (which was to be the dominant paradigm of the twentieth century), but rather on ensuring a comfortable physical environment for patients.

John Conolly's success in adapting the small-scale experiments at the York Retreat to a large institution had played an essential role in the drafting of the new 1845 Lunacy Act. From that date all new asylums were expected to follow his lead, not only in treatment but in the design and construction of buildings. In 1847, two important publications determined the structure and nature of asylums for the rest of the nineteenth century. Conolly published his influential *The Construction and Government of Asylums and Hospitals for the Insane* in which he described how building design and treatment should work together to provide humane and effective care for pauper lunatics.

In the same year, the Lunacy Commissioners produced a booklet entitled *The Further Report of the Commissioners in Lunacy*, which contained guidance about the siting and building of new asylums. The Commissioners were very prescriptive and included strict financial limits to be set by both the Commissioners themselves and the locally based Visitors' Committees. They also stipulated what sorts of sites were considered acceptable. The *Report* evolved into *Suggestions and Instructions* ('*in reference to 1. – sites, 2. – construction and arrangement of buildings, 3. – plans of lunatic asylums*') and was frequently updated to take account of advances in architectural design; these extracts are from the 1856 edition:

> The site of the building should be elevated, in respect to the surrounding countryside... cheerful in its position and having a fall to the South of the building. The building should be placed near the northern boundary of the land; and it is important that the site should afford a plateau of sufficient extent for the whole structure, and ready access from the North; the whole of the southern portion of the land being available for the undisturbed use of the patients.[21]

The asylum itself had to be built on flat, well-drained land protected from northerly winds by shelter-belts of trees. It was always intended that the new asylums should be self-sufficient, and the local Committee of Visitors were expected to plan for a farm to be part of the site. This was to be worked by staff and male patients and supply virtually all of the asylum's food. For this reason, the guidelines contained the injunction that:

> The land belonging to the asylum should, where practicable, be in proportion of not less than one acre to four patients, so as to afford ample means for agricultural employment, exercise and recreation; and that it should be so situated as to offer facilities for any extension which may become necessary at a future period.[22]

During the planning stage, the Commissioners in Lunacy had to approve three key aspects of all new asylums: the selection of the site, the layout of the buildings on the land, and the design of the building, including its cost. The Commissioners had the power to compel counties to comply with their building regulations, and the Secretary of State would not grant a licence to build unless the asylum met with the Commissioners' approval. The Commissioners were necessarily preoccupied by costs, as the large asylums were expensive to construct and were, by any standards, major public works. They were mindful too that the buildings should not be too reminiscent of large country houses which would, they felt, be intimidating to the inmates.[23] In keeping with Victorian social conventions, propriety was always a prime consideration and firm guidelines were laid out for the separation of the sexes, including the provision of separate doorways for females and males.[24]

From the 1840s, asylum building became big business and until well into the 1930s the architecture of asylums became a specialist subject in its own right. The nineteenth century was a time of innovation and, as architects solved the difficulties of designing and constructing such large-scale buildings housing up to 2000 people in an efficient and healthy way, various new ideas were tried out. The Commissioners in Lunacy ensured that each design complied with their *Suggestions and Instructions* but this did not restrict experimental design.

In the same year as the Commissioners in Lunacy first published guidance on the siting and construction of asylums, George Goodwin, the editor of the weekly magazine *The Builder*, began to publish a series of articles on the design of asylums and general hospitals.[25] He criticised plans for the then newly built Colney Hatch Asylum for being too large with 2000 inmates, and too high at three storeys. Goodwin played his part in promoting the evolution of asylum design by commissioning a series of articles by a fellow architect, Henry Burdett. Burdett categorised the plans being submitted to the Commissioners in Lunacy into four types: irregular, corridor, pavilion, or corridor-pavilion.[26] All designs, however, were expected to meet some basic criteria. They should allow for inmates with different classifications of lunacy to be treated separately, aid the supervision of patients both within the building and in the grounds, and maximise natural sunlight and free ventilation of air. There should be easy communication between different parts of the building, and the corridors should not go through sleeping, eating, working or activity areas for either staff or patients.

Burdett used these criteria to assess the relative merits of each of his four types. The irregular classification covered all asylums which had not been specifically designed as asylums but had, instead, been adapted to meet that need. Originally, most of these had been built as large country houses and had become notorious during the early part of the century as private madhouses.[27]

The vast majority of asylums designed from the 1840s to the 1870s fell into the corridor category. It was the most favoured of designs during the middle part of the nineteenth century, principally because it fulfilled the rule that people did not have to go through wards or working areas when moving about the building. Three Counties Asylum was to be a notable example of the corridor type. Its architect, George Fowler Jones, had tried to make his long corridors reminiscent of the Elizabethan and Jacobean long rooms, which were a feature in great houses. Indeed, the 1856 plans for TCA show these corridors radiating out from the central core to the male and female sides, well lit by windows ranged along their length.[28] The best type of corridor design had rooms on one side of the corridor only. Those with rooms on both were considered badly ventilated and lacking sufficient light. During the 1850s and 1860s, there were some eighteen county and five borough asylums built, all using various types of corridor design.

As asylums began to cater for upwards of 1,000 patients, the limitations of trying to house them all in a single building that did not look entirely institutional began to create problems. This was especially the case because of the strict budget set by the Commissioners. The logical solution was a pavilion or villa design with detached wards to house the more able-bodied patients, who could then lead semi-independent lives. This would dispense with the long corridors and make the asylum look more like a small village. Unfortunately, it proved to be impractical with such large numbers of patients requiring institutional care, and it was not recommended for county asylums.

From the mid-1880s the corridor-pavilion design was promoted by both Burdett and the Commissioners, although it came too late to influence the original design or the two subsequent major extensions which shaped the building of the Three Counties Asylum. Essentially a cross between the corridor designs of the 1850s and the pavilion proposals, it consisted of separate buildings attached to a central block by long, well-lit corridors.

The Design of the New Asylum at Arlesey

The Lunacy Commissioners made only one initial criticism of Jones's architectural plans for the asylum.[29] They pointed out that having some entrances to the asylum on the south side of the building was contrary to their new *Suggestions and Instructions*.[30] Marlborough Pryor arranged a meeting with the Commissioners in London to discuss their criticism and took Hill and Jones with him. The Commissioners backed down, agreeing that the plans had been drawn up before the new edition had been printed, and that they were therefore unable to insist that all doorways be moved. However, they did request certain other amendments that were accepted, and the number of entrances was subsequently reduced to four while extra accommodation was to be provided near to the planned workshops and laundry.

With these amendments the plans were accepted, although the rooms near to the workshops were not actually built until the first extension of the building in 1872. The Secretary of State gave outline permission for the building in May 1856, and Jones was instructed to prepare detailed plans and specifications which were ready by 9 September.[31] Just as the Visitors' Committee were confident that building could proceed, the Commissioners came back with a further list of amendments to the plans which caused some consternation at the next Committee meeting. The Commissioners drew the Committee's attention to the following points:

1. The dormitories did not allow 48 cubic feet per patient and did not have a minimum ceiling height of eleven feet.
2. There was not complete separation of the sexes, especially at mealtimes.
3. Less than one fifth of patients were to be housed in single rooms (the recommended proportion was one third).
4. Stone lintels should be placed between the rooms to prevent the spread of fire.
5. There was insufficient provision for warming the larger rooms.
6. Ventilation was insufficient and should be improved by constructing large ducts in the walls arranged so that the heating from the fires would draw the air through.[32]

Jones wrote to the Commissioners and pointed out that the flooring, warming and ventilation he proposed were exactly as he had put into the extensions at the North and East Ridings Asylum at York, and the new asylum near Cambridge where they had raised no objection. He did concede that the dormitories were smaller than he intended, and added 'this must have been an oversight' which he would be happy to correct. The use of a single dining room where male and female staff and patients might mix was, says Fowler, the Commissioners' own suggestion, and he wondered why they did not question its inclusion in the plans at an earlier stage.

The Committee of Visitors, however, resolved that the plans must be altered to address all their criticisms, and the modifications were included in their submission to the Secretary of State. The Secretary of State gave his formal approval on 19 November 1856 and at this point invitations to tender were put out. On 9 May 1857 William Webster of Boston, Lincolnshire was awarded the contract.

Jones saw himself as being responsible for every part of the building, including decoration and furnishings. Having seen the negative effects of poor design at Colney Hatch, there is little doubt that Jones made strenuous efforts, within the financial limits set by the Commissioners, to make his design for Three Counties Asylum as cheerful and aesthetically pleasing as possible.[33] Burdett had dismissed the linear-corridor design of Colney Heath by claiming in *The Builder* that 'the asylum [at Colney Hatch] has no special feature beyond its great size. There is nothing worth imitation in its design.'[34] Jones was determined to make his design less institutional. At his first asylum at Fulbourn, Cambridgeshire, he had used curved corridors around a central building with some embellishments on the towers (which were necessary features for water storage) and detailing on the facade.

The completion of the asylum occurred in three phases, the first of which was the original main block of the building. For this Jones came up with a symmetrical plan around a central courtyard, divided by a single-storey passage at ground level. It had a single administrative block on the south side (the main entrance) which until 1936 also housed the medical superintendent. The north block contained the chapel and kitchens. To the east were the male wards and workshops, and to the west a laundry and the female wards. Jones also designed the gasworks, which were built before the main building, and the farmyard and buildings which were eventually placed to the north of the site.

Webster was clearly a resourceful man. It is noted in the Building Committee minutes, for example, that when he ran short of bricks, he excavated clay and made his own.[35] He also provided the carved-oak chimneypiece for the medical superintendent's front parlour (later the committee room) as a gift to the Visiting Committee, and a small brass plaque was attached to it recording Webster's generosity.[36]

Although the Committee had enthusiastically embraced Jones's plans for the new asylum when they were presented in 1856, as they saw the building rise they began to agitate for some changes. Much attention was given to the glazing of the windows, which had not yet been fitted. One of the Bedfordshire visitors, Francis Pym, had been to Cambridgeshire to inspect the Fulbourn project which was near completion. He observed that the brickwork and carpentry were well done but the plan of the buildings was so different from Arlesey that no proper comparisons could be made, except for a few details common to both, which were undesirable and needed altering. The most notable was the design of the windows:

> which are glazed with small panes in an iron frame. Only single frames open and they give a most melancholy aspect to the building – which is directly contrary to the cheerful appearance so essentially necessary in a lunatic asylum. Similar frames, although larger, are to be used at Arlesey but the same error exists in their mode of opening.[37]

Pryor wrote to several of the newly opened asylums asking about the windows used, the size of each pane of glass, the construction of the opening, and the size of the space that could be opened. He received replies in the form of letters, plans and suggestions from the medical superintendents of nineteen different asylums, including some observations from Mr Denne, the resident medical superintendent of Bedford.[38] The Committee, drawing on this advice, suggested to Jones that he 'make the panes used for the glazing of the windows as large as possible compatible with the security of the patients in order to produce a light appearance to the building from without and an air of cheerfulness to the patients within the asylum'.[39] Hill and Jones duly amended their design for the window frames and the size of the openings.

County asylum buildings housed a large number of patients and staff and, in the days before piped hot water for washing, it was essential that air was encouraged to circulate to reduce odours and possible contamination. Jones used his own system of ventilation which he had experimented with at Fulbourn (and which is fully described in his 1877 extension plans). Smooth vertical clay pipes were built into the walls as they were raised. The bottom of the pipe opened into the outside air and rose by the fireplace into an opening near the ceiling. The theory was that the fire would heat the air in the pipe, causing it to flow from outside to inside, ventilating the rooms without creating a draught.

Jones was convinced that his method would meet the asylum's needs and he had won over the Visitors' Committee to his point of view. However, in practice, the system appeared to be somewhat deficient, as comments recorded soon after the opening of the asylum complain of 'smells' in the wards and dayrooms. In his subsequent extensions, Jones was to abandon iron windows altogether in favour of wooden sash ones which could be fully opened when the patients were off the ward, and this appears to have been more successful in meeting the need for 'adequate and wholesome air to cleanse the rooms' which the Lunacy Commissioners demanded.[40]

Jones's design for the asylum showed a number of influences. Nicholas Bridges, an architect who gave evidence to an enquiry about a proposed housing development on the Fairfield site in 1998, noted that the asylum had:

> a pronounced Gothic influence, visible in the general massing of the building and the detailing of the windows ... at the same time the stone embellishments to the front of the superintendent's house are Flemish or Jacobethan ... as are the pierced brick balustrades over the corner projections ... The profiles of the ogival, pyramidal and steeply pitched hipped towers betray an early mediaeval French influence as well as ... [aspects of] Hatfield House not far away.[41]

This almost post-modern mixing of styles was characteristic of the time. Jones had shown himself committed to the Classical style, which looked impressive in the large-scale church building projects he worked on throughout his long career, but he was not averse to using Gothic, especially where his clients demanded something in the 'new style'.

When it came to the third phase of development at Three Counties Asylum between 1877 and 1882, Jones designed a chapel in a simple Early English Gothic style with an exceptional hammerbeam roof.

The Clock Turret

The main building as we see it today is, from the outside at least, largely unaltered from that which Jones originally completed in the third phase of development. This gave the building its long frontage, necessitated by adherence to the corridor style which formed the original building of 1860. Two features no longer surviving, though, are the original tall chimneys (removed in the 1970s) and the clock tower.

The clock turret stood above the south central block of the building, in what later became the main entrance. In Jones's original plans for the asylum of 1856 there is no suggestion of a clock tower above what was intended to be the medical superintendent's quarters.[42] It was clearly a later addition to the plans, almost certainly added at the insistence of the Visitors' Committee who felt it would lend grandeur to the building. First mention of the tower was at the Visitors' Committee meeting in March 1859, where it was 'Resolved that it be referred to Mr Jones to consider and report upon the best place for erecting a Clock Turret and the estimated expense thereof.'[43]

In July 1859 the Committee bought the clock mechanism from perhaps the most prestigious clockmakers in the country, Dent & Co in the Strand, who, that same year, installed Big Ben in the Houses of Parliament. The cost was £85, with two copper dials purchased at an additional cost of £16 16s, not including the bell.[44] The clock was to be powered by falling weights rather than a clockwork mechanism and this demanded a certain height so that it would run for eight days. The frame, according to Dent, needed to be 4ft 2ins long, 2ft 2ins wide and 4ft 10ins high. The weights needed about a 42ft fall if possible but, if not, the difference could be made up by using extra pulleys.

Dent also offered a bell to strike the hours at £50, but the Committee felt this was too expensive and looked elsewhere. In the end they bought one weighing four hundredweight (about 200 kg), costing £34 0 5d, from Messrs Mears of Whitechapel in London. Jones designed the tower to be placed over the medical superintendent's residence and it was subsequently erected there at a cost of £100 with the two dials facing north and south. By any standards, it was an unsightly addition to the elegant facade and skyline of Jones's south elevation. By 1902 it had been dismantled and the bell re-hung in the chapel-block tower.

Furnishings and Fixtures

In the year before the asylum was opened, Pryor and his committee were occupied with the essential minutiae of turning a large empty building into a functioning institution. Staff had to be engaged (see Chapter Two), furniture inspected and ordered, curtaining, tools, carpeting, and livestock purchased. The question of clothing, furniture and fittings for the new asylum was first discussed in February 1859.[45] Initially, the committee carefully looked at what they already had in the Bedford Asylum. Pryor and Pym visited some recently opened asylums at Brentwood in Essex, Leicester and Haywards Heath in Sussex. Pryor gave a rough costing for suitably outfitting the asylum for 500 patients plus staff:[46]

	£
Wards	about 2366
Clothing of patients	3960
Kitchen, larder, dairy and laundry	315
Attendants and Servants' Rooms	500

Committee Room	112
Waiting Room	5
Clerks' Offices	21
Hall	47
Superintendent's House	300
Clerk to the Visitors	20
Chaplain's Room	42
Assistant Medical Officer	42
Stewards' Apartments	70
Assistant Matron's Room	180
Storeroom	100
Surgery	100
Tools	110
Amounting to	**£8470**

At the same meeting it was agreed to ask the builder, William Webster, to build sufficient tables from 'a large stock of American Birch which he had on hand'. Pryor initially recommended that the beds also be made of the same material, 'as being the neatest and most useful, but remembering the number of iron bedsteads of a remarkable good construction recently purchased for the Bedford Asylum,' he eventually advised the committee to use these[47] but to order some wooden cots too to make up the number of beds they required.

During their annual visit in June 1859, the Commissioners were less than enthusiastic about the plans for the wooden beds. They heard that an order was being placed for 150 traditional wooden trough beds at a cost of 50/- each. The bottom of the bed was made of wood, the centre portion being lower than the rest. The mattress was designed to be divided into three parts, 'the centre portion being composed of various absorbent materials of which sponge is to form a part' – this presumably to soak up any nocturnal enuresis. Aside from their expense, the Commissioners objected strenuously to the use of old-fashioned trough beds, which were being abandoned in other asylums because metal beds were stronger (if, for example, a patient had to be restrained) as well as being easier to maintain. In the face of this censure, the committee opted for all-iron beds from Messrs Taunton and Hatton of Birmingham (who had supplied the beds for the Bedford Asylum), ordering 250 at a cost of 25/6 each.

The plan for the crockery was adapted from the Leicester Asylum: white plates with the asylum name in the centre and different-coloured plates for the use of attendants.[48] By August, the crockery design had been chosen and William Kilpin of Bedford was awarded the contract for 600 dinner plates, 600 dishes, 600 cups (without handles), 100 washing basins with ewers, 600 chamber pots (without handles) for the use of patients, 72 plates, and 60 cups and saucers with assorted beer and milk jugs, and 60 basins and ewers for attendants and servants, and a long list of dishes, glassware and cups for the 'Officers of the Asylum'. The total cost was £119 4s 8d.

Landscape and Farm

The land had been farmed from the date of purchase so that it would be ready for the first intake of patients. It also meant that the land earned money to offset the cost of raising and furnishing the new asylum.

Samuel Bailey of Southill was appointed bailiff on 15 September 1856. Within weeks of contracts being exchanged with Major Wilkinson, Bailey was instructed to begin draining and farming the land. He found it difficult to get local labour and recommended to the committee that a foreman should be appointed at 16/- per week so that he could recruit his own work force.[49] Bailey was also given £500 to purchase a team of horses, carts and agricultural equipment so that there would be a first harvest in 1857.[50]

In its first year of operation, the farm showed a profit of £833 18 7d, and Bailey was commended for his 'industry and management'.[51] There were six horses, twenty acres of turnips, oats, beans, barley and livestock. At this time, Bailey was using the old King's Farm buildings that had come with Wilkinson's land and there were calls from the committee for a new farmyard to be built closer to the asylum so that patients could walk to it with minimum supervision. This apparently simple task occupied the committee, especially Pryor, for the next two and a half years. Jones himself was to design, redesign and submit his plans without success, while the committee debated the best site. At first, the Committee were certain that they wanted the farm to the south of the new asylum so that it was sheltered and warmed by the sun. Samuel Hill pointed out that any structure on the south side would obscure the view of the patients working on the land and, therefore, it should be located on the north side. However, the rail tramway broke the narrow north strip of land into two parts as it curved in through a steep cutting to the rear of the building.

Pryor at once wrote to other asylums to see how they had decided to place their farmyards with respect to the main building. He made his recommendations in a lengthy report in November 1858, to which he attached a table showing the direction of the prevailing winds in England over the previous twelve months as compiled by the Royal Society:[52]

SW	112 days	N	16 days
NE	58 days	S	18 days
NW	50 days	W	53 days
SE	32 days	E	26 days

Pryor then quoted from replies he had had from 22 asylum resident medical superintendents including Prestwick, Hampshire, Gloucestershire and Lincolnshire, who all encouraged him to consider placing the farmyard as close to the building as possible. Pryor finished his report with the recommendation that the whole project should be sited 'ten yards to the west of the site earlier suggested'.[53] It was also decided that the bailiff's and the cowman's houses should be incorporated in the final plan, so that they were 'on the job', one house at each corner of the farmyard. The site was to be within the curve of the rail-tramway and this meant that a bridge had to be built over the cutting in order that a roadway could be made to the farmyard gate, which opened northwards away from the asylum building. An iron palisade four feet high was erected on each side of the eighteen-foot-span bridge, so that suicidal patients would not be tempted to throw themselves from the bridge onto the tramway tracks.[54] The new farmyard was built and ready for use by April 1860, some 30 months after the issue had first been debated by the committee. The old King's Farm buildings were pulled down in July 1860.[55]

The south face of the building was constructed so that it looked out over the land that the male patients would work on as farm labourers, and it was important that they were always in view. Jones's photographs of 1870 clearly show the building rising out of what was essentially a cleared field, although trees were cultivated on the north and east sides to shield the establishment from the prevailing winds.

When the Commissioners in Lunacy visited on 19 May 1859, the construction of the asylum was still proceeding and the farmyard and farm buildings had scarcely been started. However, their description gives a clear picture of the site:

> The land belonging to the institution amounts to 260 acres, and the building is placed upon the most elevated portion of it commanding extensive views in every direction. The situation is somewhat exposed but an embankment has been raised to the north and east, and trees have been thickly planted upon it.
>
> At the distance of a mile and a half there is a railway station at the village of Arlesey and from thence a branch railway has been laid down which is brought quite into the basement of the building on the north side – an excellent road from Arlesey has also been constructed. The whole of the land appears to be under cultivation and it is reported to be of good quality. The water supply is said to be abundant – but we could not learn that any accurate measurement of it had been made and it is important we think that this should be ascertained. The building is composed of white brick relieved with

red and it has a handsome and cheerful appearance. The principal front is to the south and the entrance on the north side ... the farm buildings are to the north and appear to be placed rather too near the main building. These are not yet completed but they will no doubt be convenient. No accommodation for working patients is provided in connection with them. The whole of the asylum is in a great state of forwardness. The floors are laid – the window sashes are fixed and the water closets, baths and other fittings are nearly completed.[56]

On the south side, airing courts were built so that those who could not work could sit out during the day. These were also an integral feature of the asylum system. Airing courts were mainly grass areas, one on each side for males and females, which were fenced in with tall iron railings. Jones's photographs of 1870 show that the land near to the asylum was landscaped and, during this time, ornamental trees were planted to create avenues, evergreens being much favoured. Trees planted included Wellington fir, bay and copper beech.

Phases II and III: Enlarging the Asylum

After some discussion by the Commissioners about overcrowding within the first few years of opening, the Visiting Committee decided in 1868 to extend the original building to allow for an increase of 180 patients. The plans were to include extra bed spaces and two recreation halls, one for males and one for females.[57] Jones was again commissioned to draw up the plans and he produced several designs in 1868. However, construction was held up for two years because of a water shortage. A drought over the summer of 1865 had created a severe water crisis for the asylum and Clutterbuck's wells could certainly not cope with any increase in patient numbers. In 1870 the wells were deepened to 505 feet and only then could Jones's plans be realised. An extra storey was added to the workshops on the male side and to the laundry on the female side, with extra day rooms built at the ends of both the male and female wings. Two recreation halls were also added symmetrically to the long north corridors. The additions were in place by 1871, the cost being £22,000, borne by the three counties proportionate to their bed allocation:

Beds	£8,079	(36%)
Herts	£10,441	(47%)
Hunts	£3,480	(17%)

The building could now hold 682 patients and, immediately after the second phase was completed, gave the medical superintendent some 56 spare beds which he anticipated would meet all the asylum's needs for many years to come. However, the numbers coming into asylum care around the country were rising fast. The increase in population for the Three Counties (see below) meant a rise from 18.27 new places needed per year on average over the period 1860–70 to 22.6 between 1871 and 1876. This was partly caused by the population increases but also because the incidence of mental illness appeared to be getting more common amongst the general population, rising from 19.7 per 10,000 in 1861 to 26.7 per 10,000 in 1875.[58]

	Census 1861	Census 1871	Increase
Beds	135,287	146,257	10,970
Herts	173,280	192,226	18,946
Hunts	64,250	63,708	(-542)
TOTALS	372,817	402,191	29,374

Change in Population in Bedfordshire, Hertfordshire and Huntingdonshire, 1861–1871

In a special report for the Visiting Committee in 1876, Pryor's successor, Colonel Lindsell, concluded that the counties had three choices in dealing with the overcrowding which was already apparent. Firstly, they could begin 'boarding out' patients, which meant sending patients 'who are in a fair way of recovery to the care of their friends'. These patients would remain on the books of the asylum for two months and an allowance be paid by the asylum for their maintenance at home. At the end of that period, if certified as fit for discharge, they would then be removed from the registers.[59] Alternatively, the counties could build a new asylum for 400–500 inmates, or expand the present asylum to bring its capacity up to 1000.

The recommendation of the chairman and the medical superintendent was to extend Three Counties Asylum and Jones was again asked to present plans for the further accommodation of 318 new beds. For an estimated cost of £57,000, the work was contracted and the funds made available at the Courts of Quarter Sessions in 1877. The expansion had become pressing as the Committee had found it necessary to move twenty-four patients to Ipswich Asylum because of overcrowding. In the event, the new extensions were to cost some £15,000 more than estimated by Jones but in return the Three Counties gained a large modern asylum with 1,000 beds, two isolation wards (diphtheria, scarlet fever, tuberculosis and typhoid were then common infectious diseases which required swift isolation), and a new chapel.[60]

The tramway was also extended and a new platform was built beneath the 1871 extension to the laundry. The siting of the chapel (later named St Luke's) was originally to be in the female airing court on the south side of the building, but was built to the north in the shelter of a belt of trees. It was opened in December 1879 and the rest of the new buildings opened in 1881.

Corridors running east–west were built at ground level to the north of the existing wards, to provide a route which avoided going through dormitories and wards. It was at this time that two male and two female wards were added, with new airing courts at the extreme east and west ends of the building. The extension to the east (male) side sliced through the screening trees planted in 1858. The female airing court had an original ha-ha wall which is still there (a ha-ha wall is a sloping ditch walled on the inside below ground level). This allowed patients an unobstructed view of the land to the south of the building while ensuring their custody within the yard.

The Asylum after Opening

In 1861, a year after the asylum opened, Samuel Hill, who had helped the Committee plan and organise the building of the Three Counties, was asked by the Commissioners in Lunacy in London to make the first formal progress report on the building works. The report provides a vivid description of the original asylum:

> It stands on an estate of upwards of 250 acres of elevated tablelike land, and is approached from the village of Arlesey by a bold carriage drive; running parallel to which is a tramway from the Great Northern Railway, for the transit of heavy goods, coals to the stoves, gas-works, and other engineering departments. Although the convenience of a tramway may be regarded as advantageous for the purposes specified, yet the deep cutting, as it reaches nearer to the building, cannot be altogether free from objection, on the score of the safety of patients whose maladies too frequently deprive them of self-command or control. The design may be said to consist of a double-fronted edifice, north and south, the roads already mentioned running up to the former, where is situated the great block, containing the kitchen and scullery, larder, dairy, bakehouse, bread-rooms, and other domestic offices; over which is the Chapel, a room for the Chaplain, and apartments for some of the officers. Gas is used for cooking, and the tea and coffee apparatus operates well.
>
> The carriage drive is extended round the west [female side] to the south, where the Superintendent's residence is, forming a divisional block, together with the Matron's and Steward's store-rooms, surgery, Clerk's office, Committee-room &c., &c. Over the store-rooms are the Infirmaries, and an attendant's room for each.
>
> The connexion between the north block first spoken of (comprising the domestic offices, etc.) and south central block is by

an enclosed but light and airy passage. The conveyance of food to the wards right and left, is also by covered ways, across which are means for heavy traffic. The arrangements of the wards are exceedingly simple; they are short, with corridors 12 feet wide, in which are single bed-rooms for patients, and attendants' rooms, lavatory, &c...

Leading from the Female side is a passage to the laundry, wash-houses, drying-rooms and drying-grounds. From the Male or east wing, in like manner, are placed the workshops, consisting of tailors, shoemakers, carpenters, painters and plumbers, smith's shop, and brewhouse. Independently of these buildings is a shed, at the end of which, on the Female side, is the steam-engine and boiler-house for pumping water and for steam for the laundry, and one, too, on the Male side, in the materials' yard belonging to the workshops, with an out-door store-room. The Asylum on the upper floors consists entirely of sleeping rooms.

It is built of white brick, relieved with red and black, with stone quoins in parts. The pleasure-grounds [airing courts] are on the south side, and protected on two sides by the main buildings of the Asylum, by which they are entered, by four porched doorways; iron palisades bound them. The clock tower presents a prominent object. The farm buildings lie between the main roads of approach and the workshops; they are very commodious, and embrace every requisite convenience and accommodation for live as well as dead stock. The bailiff's house and a couple of cottages adjoin, and there is also a block of four cottages across the Stotfold Road for the families of servants employed on the premises. There is also a Chaplain's residence and a lodge [down the Arlesey Drive]. The plan is capable of extension, both by raising the whole a second floor, and by adding onto the extreme east and west wings.[61]

Initially, there was no set date for the new asylum to receive its first patients and it was decided in June 1859 that it should be postponed until as early as possible in the new year.[62] However, with the Commissioners in Lunacy in London urging haste, by January 1860 the Committee were putting pressure on Webster and Jones to finish. At a meeting on Monday 20 February 1860, Jones was able to say that he 'fully expected the building would be completed by the contractor to give over to the committee on 5 March next'.[63] A meeting was called to conduct the handover. However, by 5 March there had been delays and Jones reported that there were several little things to do before he could certify the completion of the asylum, and the handover had to be postponed for another two weeks.[64] At the meeting of 19 March 1860 it was noted that Jones had delivered a report certifying that the buildings and works were complete and ready to receive patients. The Visitors then declared the asylum 'erected pursuant to the Lunatic Asylums Act 1853 to be so far completed as to be fit for the reception of Pauper Lunatics from the united counties and from the Borough of Bedford ... and that after the second day of April next the asylum be opened for the reception of patients generally' (although the first group of patients had been transferred from the Bedford Asylum on 8 March). They further ordered that notices of the opening be put in the county newspapers, and requested all Clerks of the Boards of Guardians to submit the names of all pauper lunatics belonging to the counties but resident in asylums outside the area so that they might be transferred to Three Counties Asylum.

Notes

1   B. Cashman, *A Proper House: Bedford Lunatic Asylum 1812–1860*. North Bedfordshire Health Authority 1992.
2   Cashman, 1992, 104.
3   Bedfordshire Quarter Sessions, 1856.
4   LF55/1, Agreement to Unite so far as Provision for Lunatics was Concerned, 15 Dec 1855.
5   LF4/5/1, Minutes of Committee for Providing New Asylum, 28 Jan 1856.
6   *Ibid.*, 21 Feb 1856.
7   *Ibid.*
8   *Ibid.*, 10 Mar 1856.
9   LF4/5/1.
10   LF4/5/1, 28 Jul 1856.
11   N. Bridges, Evidence to Enquiry on Proposed Redevelopment of Fairfield Hospital – Appendix NB/F & NB/C, 1998.
12   LF4/5/1, Jun 1856.
13   *Ibid.*, 24 Oct 1856.
14   *Ibid.*, 11 May 1857.
15   LF4/6/1, Minutes of the Building Committee, 12 Jun 1857.
16   *Ibid.*, J. Clutterbuck, Report to the Building Committee, 1857.
17   K. Jones, *Asylums and After. A Revised History of the Mental Health Services from the Early 18th Century to the 1990s*. Athlone Press 1993, 26–33.
18   *Ibid.*, 36–7.
19   Cashman, 1992.
20   The Lunacy Act, 1845 (8 & 9 Vict. c100 & c126).
21   LF4/5/3, 'Suggestions and Instructions in Reference to Lunatic Asylums', HMSO 1856.
22   *Ibid.*
23   *Ibid.*
24   *Ibid.*
25   H. Burdett, *The Builder*, 1847.
26   H. Burdett, *Hospitals and Asylums of the World*, J & A Churchill, London 1891, 59–61.
27   *Ibid.*, Vol. 1, 59–60.
28   These were demolished in the second phase of building in 1871 and the new corridors were much less attractive and allowed for very little natural light.
29   LF4/5/1, 20 Mar 1856.

30   LF4/5/3, Section 2.2.

31   LF4/5/1, May 1856.

32   *Ibid.*, 17 Nov 1856.

33   Surviving records of each stage of the construction of the Three Counties
      Asylum are remarkably complete and detailed. The two principle sources for
      the architectural record are 'Minutes of the Commissioners of Justices and
      Visitors, 1855–1858' and the 'Building Committee Minutes Book 1855–1860'
      Although these include a large number of plans and some wash drawings
      all signed by Jones, a more complete set was found by Nicholas Bridges at
      the Public Record Office which houses the architectural archives of the
      Commissioners in Lunacy.

34   Burdett 1847, 586.

35   LF1/1, 20 Sept 1859.

36   The chimneypiece was stolen in November 1997 from the empty hospital
      building.

37   LF4/5/1, 22 Feb 1858.

38   *Ibid.*

39   *Ibid.*

40   LF4/5/3.

41   N. Bridges, op. cit.

42   This part of the building remained the medical superintendent's residence from
      1860 until the 1930s when Icknield House was built nearby.

43   LF1/1, 21 Mar 1859.

44   *Ibid.*, 18 Jul 1859.

45   *Ibid.*, Feb 1859.

46   *Ibid.*

47   *Ibid.*, 21 Mar 1859.

48   *Ibid.*

49   LF/4/5/1.

50   *Ibid.*, Jan 1857.

51   *Ibid.*

52   LF4/5/1, 29 Nov 1858.

53   *Ibid.*

54   The cutting was filled in when the tramway was taken up in the 1950s.

55   LF1/1.

56   LF1/1, 19 May 1859.

57   LF1/3, 1868.

58   LF1/5, 1875. The increase in asylum admission rates is contested within the
      history of psychiatry. For example, see A. Scull, 'Was insanity increasing? A
      response to Edward Hare.' *British Journal of Psychiatry*, 144, 1984, 432–6.

59   LF1/5, 25 Aug 1876.

60   The Isolation Hospital built to the north of the hospital became, in the 1920s,
      the nurses' home and, from 1948, the Nurse Training School. It was closed in
      1990. The Isolation Hospital is interesting because it is built on a butterfly plan,
      having a central block rising higher than the two wings.

61   LF1/1. This pavilion or villa style of development suggested by Hill was not
      taken up until the 1930s when the Fairfield Admissions Unit was built, along
      with two villa wards. The eventual extensions to the asylum made in the 1870s
      were added to the main building itself.

62   LF1/1, Jun 1859.

63   *Ibid.*, 20 Feb 1860.

64   *Ibid.*, 5 Mar 1860.

CHAPTER TWO

The Social Landscape
of a Victorian Asylum

On 8 March 1860, the new Three Counties Asylum admitted its first patients, six men and six women transferred from the Bedford Asylum. Only the sketchiest details survive about what life was like for those patients transferred to the new asylum. Nevertheless, we will attempt to give a flavour of daily life in the early years of the institution, both internally – what it was like to live and work in the asylum – and externally – its connections to the broader community and how it operated within the constraints of regulatory agencies. To do this we have looked primarily at the social relations of groups at all levels of the institution – patients, staff, administration, governing bodies, clergy and community residents. To understand the types of illnesses and life circumstances that brought patients to the asylum in the nineteenth century (often substantially different from twenty-first-century diagnoses) we first look at the context of insanity in mid-Victorian England.

Moral and Medical Treatment

Lunacy reformers of the early and mid-nineteenth century emphasised that the asylum was to be a place of treatment. The mentally ill were to be confined in an attempt to treat them and then returned to society. The approach to be used was that of 'moral treatment', which had been pioneered at the York Retreat. Moral treatment emphasised the role of the environment as the prime therapeutic tool. The asylum was to provide a safe and comfortable environment where the mentally ill could be treated in a humane way and actively assisted to recover. When the Three Counties Asylum opened, moral treatment remained an ideal, but a largely unattainable one. In reality, treatment in the Victorian asylum was minimal. Year after year the Lunacy Commissioners – the official 'watchdogs' of asylum care – had to acknowledge in their annual reports that the majority of asylum patients did not recover.[1]

In the 1840s and early 1850s, the Commissioners focused their attention on curative issues. In 1847 they brought out a survey of treatment techniques currently in use in asylums in the hope of stimulating further advances. Results were not forthcoming and the Commissioners turned their attention to administrative matters. By the mid-1850s, the success of an asylum in curing its inmates ranked considerably below such issues as the composition of the inmates' soup.[2]

The Commissioners' annual reports show clearly that a good asylum was one in which the bedding was 'clean and sufficient', the treatment 'humane and judicious', the patients 'orderly, free from excitement and satisfactorily clothed' and the institution 'clean and tidy', attendance at chapel high, mortality rates low and the entire place efficient and industrious.[3] Asylum doctors were praised for their administrative abilities, their 'kindliness' and their perceived ability to make their patients comfortable. There was much emphasis on required paperwork and none on therapeutic initiatives, particularly those which might involve the risk of patients absconding or committing suicide. While the intention was to prevent the abuses of an earlier era, it was a stifling system which encouraged a monotonous and paternalistic environment where simply keeping patients alive became an end in itself.

At TCA the lack of medical treatment available in the 1860s is evidenced by the absence of any comments on treatment in the annual reports. The first annual report, for example, notes merely that while a padded room existed, no means of restraint were in use in the asylum.[4] 'Restraint' in this context refers to mechanical restraint: the chains and manacles which were standard features of earlier asylum treatment. Seclusion and physical restraint were used in TCA and the rules and regulations published in 1878 provided clear guidelines for their use:

> No instrument of restraint shall be placed on any patient: and no patient shall be restrained or secluded at any time, except by medical authority, and the same be recorded in the Medical Journal and Case Book; and no forcible means shall be used for giving food or medicine, except in the presence of one of the Medical Officers, or of the Head-attendant in each division.[5]

Restraint was necessary on occasions but used much more rarely than before the change in the law in 1845. Patients were usually restrained to their beds by wrapping the sheets tightly round the person and securing them to the bed-frame or, if this were not enough, leather straps might be employed or a strait-waistcoat (also sometimes referred to as a strait-jacket). Hence the need for strong iron beds rather than wooden ones. In all cases the use of restraint had to be entered into the hospital's record book and made available to the Visitors' Committee at their regular inspections.[6]

The medical superintendent's report for February 1878 outlined the approach to treatment in the asylum:

> The treatment of the patients has consisted principally in improving their health by good food, producing sleep in the sleepless (a large contingent among the newly admitted), and trying to induce them to forget their troubles by employment, amusement, etc. For producing sleep, moderate doses of chloral or hyoscyamine, with bromide of potassium are found the most effective measures we possess.[7]

The Asylum in the Community

The building of an asylum in a rural area had a significant impact on the local landscape and population. The large Victorian asylum not only dominated the skyline but played a major role in the life of the people who lived in the surrounding villages. Situated between the villages of Arlesey and Stotfold, Three Counties Asylum had a transformative effect on community life from its inception. Large numbers of villagers were employed in the institution and in some cases it provided jobs for generations of families. For those not immediately associated with the asylum, its presence was nevertheless felt in a variety of ways. It provided a source of income for local tradespeople, a place where entertainment, sporting activities and festivals took place, a place to take a shortcut through, a place to fear, and it was the object of local stories, myths and gossip.

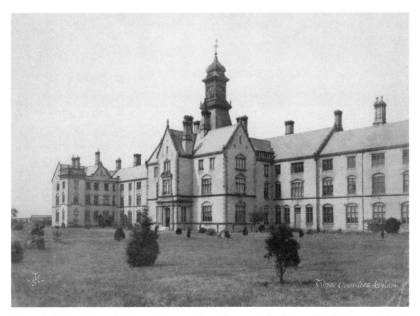

Figure 2.1 South front showing clock tower, from photograph by George Fowler Jones, c. 1870

The social life of the asylum extended beyond the neighbouring villages to the major towns of Bedfordshire, Hertfordshire and Huntingdonshire. The local landowners, clergy, businessmen and magistrates of these urban centres formed the backbone of the Visiting Committee which oversaw the running of the asylum (under the 1845 Lunacy Act they were obliged to make unannounced visits to the asylum around six times a year to check on conditions and so forth). Committee members, all men initially, were responsible for every aspect of asylum life. No matter was too small to escape their watchful attention. Their reports form the basis of the formal record of the institution and record most of what we know about daily life at TCA in the nineteenth and early twentieth centuries.

Like the dignitaries, the patients were also local residents, but much less privileged ones. They were villagers and townspeople who worked the land, laboured, served as domestics or worked in local trades or crafts. With the exception of a very small number of private patients, local people were admitted to the asylum under the category of 'pauper lunatics': members of the public who could not afford to pay the cost of their treatment.

This local world of the asylum extended beyond to the official regulatory body, the Commissioners in Lunacy. The Commissioners were eminent members of the public who had themselves often been involved in the care of the mentally ill. The Commissioners inspected every asylum on a yearly basis and wrote their all-important report detailing both strengths and criticisms. Their suggestions were taken seriously and implemented as far as possible, for they would be checked for compliance the following year.

The social network of the asylum included many groups who had a greater or lesser interest in its operation. Besides patients, staff and local community members, these included the medical establishment, which was struggling to establish its primacy as the most appropriate profession to treat the insane, patients' relatives and friends, interested social reformers, the clergy, local officials, government and the public. It took the combined efforts of all these groups over a decade from conception to opening to ready the new asylum to receive its first patients.

Arriving at the Asylum

The first group of twelve patients from Bedford Asylum ranged in age from 27 to 77 and their history of hospitalisation from seven weeks to 34 years. The oldest member of the group, F.H., aged 77, had been mentally ill for 34 years whereas 48-year-old S.B. had been ill for just seven weeks. We do not know what the selection criteria for this first group were, but it is notable that the group included two men and two women from each of the three participating counties (Hertfordshire, Bedfordshire and Huntingdonshire).

No description remains of how the patients transferred from the Bedford Asylum, but we know that they travelled by train to Arlesey. The Committee of Visitors' Annual Report for 1860 notes that the Committee 'were much indebted to the authorities of the Midland and Great Northern Railway Companies for the assistance they rendered'.[8] It is not known how they got from Arlesey station to TCA – possibly they walked or travelled by carriage, as there is no record of the asylum tramway having been used for anything other than transporting materials.

The lack of press coverage of the arrival of the first patients is due either to its coinciding with a high-profile local murder trial or to the Justices' and Committee of Visitors' deliberate decision to keep the transfer of large numbers of mentally ill people out of the media.[9] The arrival of the first patients at Fulbourn Asylum in Cambridge two years earlier may have presented a similar scene. It was described by the *Cambridge Chronicle*:

> Lunatic-Asylum Visitors met at the Asylum on Tuesday last. The main object of the meeting was to open the asylum for the reception of patients, Dr Bryan having been instructed to remove from the Hoxton Asylum the patients chargeable to Cambridge parishes on this day; accordingly shortly after the Visitors had commenced the business of the meeting, the porter announced the arrival of the train containing the poor unfortunates. Nothing could exceed the good arrangements made for removing the patients, by which all had arrived safely and without a single casualty. With the exception of three (who were carried) all walked from the carriages to the Asylum. It was a sad sight to witness, forty-six poor creatures, varying from sixteen to at least seventy years of age, each bearing the unmistakable impress of insanity. We understand several of the patients were very violent cases; but whether from their being accompanied by their own attendants, or from the change of scene, all were quiet and behaved well; in fact several of them took off their hats to the Visitors, and the females curtsied. There were about an equal number of each sex in the forty-six patients. Several of the females were very lively, and laughed heartily on walking across the grounds of the asylum.[10]

While the transfer of the Bedford Asylum patients to the Three Counties Asylum is not recorded, the new medical superintendent William Denne was praised for the 'masterly way in which he had produced order and regularity from a state of chaos' by the Justices at the midsummer Quarter Sessions, suggesting that the transfer process was not easy. It seems also to have taken a toll on the health of the patients as the Visitors' end-of-year report for 1860 suggests that the high number of deaths (37) that had occurred in the first year were 'caused most probably by the excitement consequent upon the removal'.[11]

First Patients

Nineteenth-century case notes for individual patients were very sketchy and poorly kept. Large general ledgers were used, which followed on from year to year, making it difficult to trace case histories of individuals. Most notations consisted of a phrase or two recorded annually or semi-annually about the general health of the patient. Admission registers, however, were meticulously kept, as they formed the basis for the statistical data for the annual reports and for charging the counties for patient maintenance. Thus, there is a large amount of statistical data for official purposes, but very little qualitative and descriptive material on the lives of those who populated the asylum.

The first patient to be admitted to the newly opened asylum was F.H., a 77-year-old single man from Toddington, Bedfordshire. The Admissions Register states that F.H. suffered from mania with delusions and while he had been mentally ill for 34 years, he was in good physical health.[12] F.H. remained at TCA for the rest of his life and worked on the hospital farm until well into his nineties. Case notes for 1883 describe F.H. as rarely speaking to anyone. He liked 'to sit on the ground in all weathers in preference to a seat'. Although he was feeble, by now unable to work and classified as demented, he was considered to be in good general health. In 1885 he was reported as being paralysed on his right side and weaker, necessitating his confinement to bed, though he was still in a fair condition. By the spring of 1886 he could no longer get up and a final entry in June states that he was 'slowly sinking'. F.H. died at TCA in June 1886 aged 103, twenty-six years after he became its first patient.

The first female patient to be admitted to TCA was H.C. At the time of her admission, H.C. was a 56-year-old widow who was formerly a domestic servant from North Mymms, Hertfordshire. The Register states that she was melancholic, pale but in good physical health, and had been ill for three years. H.C. recovered and was discharged in September 1860. She was readmitted, however, in August 1864 in a 'state of mania with delusions and was expected to be suicidal ... the cause of her insanity is said to be loss of family'. After a second discharge she reappears again in 1871, admitted as a washerwoman from the Hatfield workhouse. In 1875 she was working a mangle in the asylum laundry and was described as quiet and industrious. By 1878 she was unable to work, being alternately overexcited and not speaking for days, suffering from various delusions such as her children being killed. By 1884 she had become demented and noisy, in feeble health. Two years later she was described as rather depressed and full of delusions. She died in the asylum in 1889 aged 84 and was buried in the asylum burial grounds.[13]

This first group also included S.B., a 48-year-old married labourer from Wellingborough. S.B.'s diagnosis was mania with delusions. The 'Supposed Cause of Insanity' section of the Admissions Register, which was frequently left blank, recorded that S.B.'s insanity was hereditary. He had been unwell for thirteen months and had had a previous attack three years earlier. S.B.'s stay at TCA was brief and on 28 April 1860 he became one of the first patients to be discharged.[14]

K.B. was a 33-year-old dressmaker from Ayot St Peter in Hertfordshire. She was single, in good physical health and diagnosed as suffering from melancholia and delusions for twelve years. The cause of her insanity was listed as 'religious ecstasy'. Although K.B. remained in the hospital for many years, we discover little about her other than that she was a 'regular and industrious laundry worker'. In 1897 she died in the asylum at the age of 70 and was buried in the asylum burial ground.[15]

J.H. was admitted as a 30-year-old unmarried woman from Godmanchester who worked as a domestic servant. She was diagnosed as suffering from mania, her general health was good but she was 'subject to occasional attacks of hysteria when she was violent and destructive'. She had been ill for three years. She worked in the hall and, according to the case notes, she sometimes 'behaves in an indescribable insane manner, appears to be demented: but knows all passing around ... is very peculiar'. In 1878 she was recorded as being 'spiteful at times: makes many false extravagant statements such as that her arm or leg is broken'. She continued to work on a daily basis in the hall. She too died and was buried in the asylum in 1889.[16]

S.R. was a 49-year-old single labourer who had been ill for thirteen months prior to his transfer to TCA. This was his second 'attack of insanity', the first having occurred three years previously. He was suffering from mania with delusions. The frequent complaint of the Commissioners in Lunacy during TCA's early years that case notes were erratically kept is particularly apt in this case. Ten years elapsed between S.R.'s admission and the second entry which notes that S.R. 'talks a good deal to himself, uses very foul language at times, works in [the] garden, health good'. Subsequent reports note that there is 'no change' in his condition and in 1881 we are told that S.R., who continued to work out of doors, became very excited and noisy at times. He had an attack of diarrhoea in 1882 and was ill for five days during which he was treated with 'opium, lead and other astringents'. He continued to work in the garden throughout the 1880s and had 'many delusions', including the belief that he owned TCA and was married to Queen Victoria.

The first small group of twelve patients had the entire asylum to themselves for a week. No descriptions remain of what they thought of their new surroundings or of their experiences of the first days of the asylum. Possibly some of the group had been on the previous visit organised by the Rev. Edward Swann, chaplain at the Bedford Asylum, for patients who were to be transferred. The responses of this group of patients, while mostly positive, were not unanimous. The report in the Chaplain's Journal for July 1859 notes that:

> A party of 10 patients were taken this week to view the new Asylum at Arlesey. They were highly delighted and have told me their opinion of the Chapel and the new arrangements. Some seem to think it will be a most complete and cheerful residence. One woman said that she thought the effect on the patients would be most salutary; another said it would be dull, there would be no society for it was a long way from any town.[17]

Beyond this comment we have no idea what the transferred patients and staff of the Bedford Asylum thought about their relocation to the countryside. Nor do we know how their relatives and friends felt about travelling to Arlesey to visit them.

First Staff Members

The first employees of the asylum were those who built it – the workmen used by the builder William Webster. They appear to have done a good job as the building sub-committee recommended in 1858 that:

> the workmen be provided with an entertainment for themselves and their wives on the occasion of the raising of the roof and for the general good conduct and that the Clerk be requested to make the necessary arrangements for carrying this order into effect under the direction of the Chairman.[18]

The entertainment, for an unspecified number of workers and their wives, took place on 20 September 1858 at a cost of:

	£	s	d
Provisions	38	2	0
Ale, porter etc.	12	11	0
Sundries	2	0	6
£	**52**	**13**	**6**

Unfortunately we do not have a description of the party but it was reported at the November building sub-committee meeting that the entertainment 'went off most satisfactorily'.[19]

In 1859 the Visitors turned their attention to the selection of staff for the new asylum. A number of the Bedford staff were transferred to TCA. William Denne was appointed resident medical superintendent and his wife, Lucy Denne, was appointed matron. Denne was the ex-Superintendent of the Bedford Asylum, and his wife its former matron. Denne's qualifications are unknown, but as he was always addressed as 'Mr' rather than 'Dr' it was likely he was not a physician. He would, however, have had some form of recognised medical qualification. Mrs Denne probably learnt her skills on the wards and from her husband as there were no qualifications for psychiatric nurses in the mid-nineteenth century. The terms of Denne's appointment to Bedford Asylum included the employment of his wife as matron. Women like Lucy Denne combined work with marriage and child-rearing and were also expected to play the social role of superintendent's wife at numerous society functions.

The Dennes had worked at the old asylum since 1854, where they had been popular employees. They had both played an important role in the final elimination of all forms of regular physical restraint, despite opposition from some members of staff.[20] In practice restraint was sometimes necessary and the asylum kept strait-waistcoats and secluded rooms on the wards where particularly violent patients could be held for short periods. However the Committee of Visitors and Justices were especially impressed with Denne's management abilities and with the improvements that he suggested and implemented at the old asylum. Visitor Henry Littledale attributed the atmosphere of 'cheerfulness and satisfaction' that he noticed among the female patients to the repairs to the rocking-horses which had been initiated by Mr Denne.

Denne served as medical superintendent until 1874, when he retired due to ill health (he was succeeded by Dr Edward Swain who had been medical officer at Brookwood Asylum near Birmingham for six and a half years). The new steward, John Barnes, was also an ex-employee of the old asylum in Bedford, as was Samuel Wing, clerk to the Committee of Visitors and Justices. John Drury was appointed assistant medical officer and the Rev. James Acton Butt as chaplain.

These appointments were made some twelve months before the Three Counties admitted its first patients. Denne was given a salary of £500 per year plus a furnished house (within the asylum building) and an allowance for coal, gas and washing. The contract specified that Denne must provide his own linen, china and domestic servants. Lucy Denne was to be paid £100 per year for her work as Matron.

The Committee of Visitors felt that they required the services of a medical man at an early stage 'in order that they may have the benefit of his advice and assistance in rendering the asylum fit for the reception of patients' prior to opening. The duties of the medical superintendent were diverse but he (the post was always held by men) was expected to be the moving force behind the day-to-day running of the asylum, having ultimate responsibility to hire, fire, and dictate to the staff how they should lead their lives. He was also expected to be a godfearing man and the Rules and Regulations for both the Bedford and the new Three Counties Asylum specified that 'as far as possible and consistent with the performance of their duties, the medical superintendent, all officers and servants should punctually attend divine Service in the Chapel'.[21]

Denne was to be responsible for the general supervision and condition of the patients and staff, and be accountable to the Committee for the management of the asylum. The Rules and Regulations also confirmed the role of the medical superintendent at the top of the management hierarchy in controlling of the affairs of the establishment: 'he shall have direction of the medical, surgical and moral treatment of the patients and superintend the performance of the duties of the matron, steward, attendants and servants'.[22]

The matron was expected not only to supervise the female nursing care offered at the asylum, but also to ensure that the housekeeping duties were smoothly run, from food preparation and serving to the cleaning of the wards and clothing. In addition, 'she should also obey the medical superintendent in all matters relating to medical care and treatment of female patients.'[23]

The next appointment, made on 26 September 1859, was that of Samuel Wing as clerk both to the new asylum and the Visitors' Committee at a salary of £200 per year plus £25 for travel. Wing had been the Clerk of the Bedford Asylum since 1848, taking control of all the day-to-day finances of the establishment. He scrutinised the household expenses and kept track of things through some twenty books and ledgers which the Lunacy Commissioners deemed essential for proper financial management.[24]

Another Bedford Asylum officer, John Barnes, was appointed steward and bailiff on the same day at a salary of £200 per year with an unfurnished house, plus 'vegetables, coals and gas'. Barnes asked that he also be allowed 'washing and milk' at the new asylum. After due consideration, the Visiting Committee in October 1859 decided that 'Mr Barnes be allowed his washing but no allowance for milk'.[25] The steward was responsible for all asylum servants and their wages and for monitoring the purchase, production and consumption of all foods and provisions, including fuels. As bailiff, Barnes also had to oversee the running of the farm.

The Three Counties also required nurses and attendants in preparation for the first intake of patients, and in November 1859 Elizabeth Webb was taken on from Bedford Asylum as the assistant matron at a salary of £30 per year, plus ten female attendants at £16 per year and two night attendants at the same salary. The head male attendant position was advertised at £35 per year, and twelve day and two night attendants at £29 per year. The asylum was built for 505 patients, which means that there was roughly one attendant to 23 inmates during the day, and one to 126 inmates at night.

A lodge porter was also taken on at £30 per year, a tailor at 12/- per week, and a shoemaker at the same wage. A gardener and under-gardener were appointed with board, lodging and washing at £35 and £24 per year (the position being given to the appropriately named Mr Gardener and Mr Cherry respectively, both from the Bedford Asylum). A brewer, baker, four outside attendants (to supervise work parties), an engineer, a gasman and a carpenter were also sought, plus a gatekeeper for the Arlesey Lodge and gate.

In January 1860, Dr John Drury MRCS was given the post of assistant medical officer at £80 per year including accommodation and washing. The employee roll call noted in the minutes of the Visiting Committee a year after Three Counties Asylum had opened its doors lists 61 members of staff.[26] These are all listed by name from Denne (at £500 per year) through to Samuel Winters, a general labourer earning 8/- per week. Included too are a blacksmith, steam engineer, coal porter, cowman, pigman and dairymaid.

Changes to personnel, however, soon occurred and Drury, the assistant medical officer, began 1861 with a series of leaves of absence and finally tendered his resignation on 25 March 1861.[27] At the same time, John Barnes was stripped of the office of bailiff by the Committee although he was to remain as steward. The reason appears to be that since the handover of the farm by Samuel Bailey in May 1860, it had shown an indifferent profit. The Visiting Committee's expectation that the farm should not only supply the dietary needs of the asylum patients and workers but show a net profit at the end of the year as well was to lead to a number of confrontations with various farm bailiffs over the next 100 years.

The remainder of the staff of the new asylum included male and female attendants, kitchen staff, farm workers and the brewer. Many were the first generation of families from the nearby villages of Arlesey and Stotfold who would provide staff for the asylum for the next 139 years.

A chaplain was to be hired at a salary of £200 including a rent-free house, whose duties meant that he 'shall devote all his time and attention to the inmates of the asylum'. Advertisements were put out in the *Ecclesiastical Gazette*, the *Clerical Journal* and the *Manchester Guardian* while Webster, the builder, was instructed to consider the cost of constructing the chaplain's house.[28] Interviews were held at the Euston Hotel in London in December 1859 in front of eight people, including Lord Charles Russell (a supporter of lunacy reform, a Whig and a friend of the Whitbread family). From a shortlist of eight (from 80 hopefuls) they elected the Rev. James Acton Butt of Skeyton, Norfolk by a show of hands. Butt took up his duties in February of 1860. The new house on the Arlesey drive was apparently not ready for him to move into when he arrived, as he was charged 14/- a week while he resided in rooms in the hospital.

The chaplain to the Bedford Asylum, Edward Swann, had hoped to move to TCA at the same time as the Dennes, Wing and Barnes, but his application was never shortlisted. When the position was advertised in October 1859 he wrote to the Visitors requesting information. The duties of the post were described as:

> two full services on the Sunday, morning prayers in the week days and daily visits to the patients, as well as performing the burial service over those who die in the asylum. I enclose a list of the Visitors but personal canvassing will not be countenanced. The house will be about half a mile from the asylum and is situated near the Great Northern Railway.[29]

Marlborough Pryor observed dryly in a letter to a friend, 'I do not think that Mr Swann has any cause for complaint for we never proposed to transfer the officers from one asylum to the other.'[30] Perhaps not, but the majority of the first staff at the new building were to be ex-Bedford Asylum employees.

The asylum chaplain was an important senior member of the staff whose status can be illustrated by the fact that he was assigned a house on site. In addition to holding regular services, the chaplain had to visit all the patients regularly and talk to them, pray with them and read to them. He kept a journal of his activities which was inspected at the monthly committee meetings and also contributed a section to the annual report. The manner in which he carried out his duties and the numbers in his congregation are regularly commented on in the monthly Visitors' reports, and in the yearly reports of the Commissioners in Lunacy. In their first report the Commissioners noted that the chaplain took prayers on a daily basis and occasionally held bible classes. The conduct of the patients at these activities was apparently 'very orderly'. The Commissioners suggested that the Rev. Acton Butt should organise schools where patients could be given some elementary instruction.[31]

By 1862 the Rev. Butt was organising singing classes in the chapel on Sundays which as many as 113 patients attended. At the Three Counties an additional responsibility of the chaplain was to look after the library – a duty that the hospital chaplains retained up until the mid-twentieth century, despite the advice from the Commissioners in Lunacy in 1865 that this responsibility should be handed over to the wards.

In general hospitals, the chapel was an optional space. In the post-1845 asylum, however, the chapel was a standard architectural feature which was required by the Commissioners in Lunacy.[32] The general planning requirements of hospital chapel design, such as a link to the main circulation-route system and ease of access for inmates, staff and visitors, also applied to the design of asylum chapels. The main difference lay in the size of the chapel. By the 1880s asylum chapels were recommended to be able to hold at least three-quarters of the patients. Revised recommendations published by the Commissioners in 1911 had changed little and emphasised that three-fifths of the patients should be able to be accommodated. Further specifications were detailed:

> It should have the usual character and arrangement of a church, and contain no special or peculiar provision for the separation of the sexes, except distinct entrances. Small closed porches or lobbies should be conveniently placed, to which epileptic patients seized by fits during services may be removed. The building, while being designed on ecclesiastical lines, must not be ornate in detail, or constructed with elaborate stonework.[33]

What was less clear was whether the chapel should be integrated within the asylum or a free-standing building in the grounds. Taylor suggests that, by 1870, the Commissioners indicated that the chapel should be in the grounds to give 'the inmates the opportunity of a walk to and from the services'.[34] Furthermore, it was felt that if the chapel was in the grounds, the inmates might 'forget' that they were in an asylum. Opponents of this approach argued that it was highly unlikely that patients would forget where they were and that a chapel should be attached to the main building

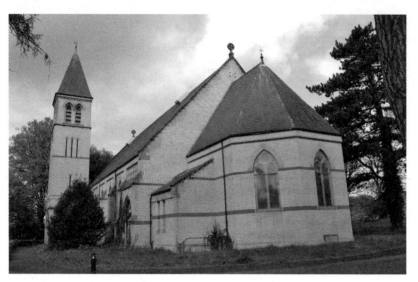

Figure 2.2 St Luke's chapel built 1878

for ease of access, greater utilisation, and to overcome the problems of bad weather. Both designs were adopted during the nineteenth century but by the early 1900s, when the villa style of building became popular, most asylum chapels were built in the grounds.

Chapel asylums were used solely for Church of England services but were not always consecrated, although the burial grounds were. This enabled the chapel space to be re-used if new and larger chapels were needed or if building plans changed. The original chapel at the Three Counties Asylum was located in the main building on the first floor. A later chapel was built in the grounds in 1879; it was consecrated and named St Luke's. Ministers of religions other than the Church of England were allowed to visit any patient who requested their services unless the medical superintendent deemed it detrimental to the health of the patient.

Social Life of the Asylum

In 1860, patients and visitors entered the asylum grounds through the newly opened entrance off Arlesey High Street. Behind the elaborately decorated wrought-iron gate a long drive led up to the main buildings. The fields on either side of the drive were part of the asylum farm and, on an average day, working parties consisting of male patients supervised by attendants could be seen cultivating the land. Part way up the drive the new arrival would pass the chaplain's house. As they neared the top of the drive the spacious and carefully laid out grounds would become visible. As the final bends in the road were negotiated, the large impressive exterior of the asylum would come fully into sight.

No descriptions or photographs survive of the interior of the asylum in the 1860s. However, the general appearance would have been similar to all county asylums of that era. There would have been distemper on the walls of the rooms, and corridors, stairways and lavatories would have been limewashed. Floors were bare pine boards with a few rugs and the stairways were concrete. All lighting was provided by gas lamps which emitted a continuous hissing sound. The rooms were stuffy and, with the gas lamps, proper ventilation was to prove a constant problem. Originally the window casements were iron but after 1880 timber sashes were used. Windows would have wooden shutters. Lavatories and bathrooms were unheated. Baths were made of lead set in five-sided wooden boxes; hot water, provided by steam boilers, was difficult to control and caps were put over taps. There was a constant hum of activity with the noise of boots on bare boards from the comings and goings of staff. The room where the Committee of Visitors held their monthly meetings would have been wallpapered and decorated and furnished in a style similar to a middle-class London home.[35]

A Visitors' report for 1860 reports that the patients 'appeared much to enjoy the light airy rooms as compared with the old asylum and many of them expressed themselves very strongly upon the subject'.[36] In their first report on the asylum a month after its opening, the Commissioners claimed that the patients' 'removal to the more cheerful wards of this building has had a beneficial effect'.[37] In this report on their initial inspection of the asylum the Commissioners provide some details of the amenities of the building:

> We have gone over all the wards and personally examined every patient … The institution has been opened so short a time that a complete organisation of the various departments cannot of course be expected. Much progress has however been made with the building and the wards are clean and in good order. The beds and bedding are of a very good description and we are glad to hear that Mr Denne intends gradually [to] discontinue the use of straw mattresses. The general furniture is still scanty but all that has been supplied is of very good quality.[38]

The use of straw mattresses remained an ongoing cause for concern. In 1865 the Commissioners commented that while the appearance of the wards had improved there were too many beds and, in particular, too many straw mattresses. Straw pillows, which were also in abundance, 'should not be used'.[39] In 1868, the Commissioners referred again to 'bedding problems' as there were approximately 90 straw mattresses in use on both the female and male sides. They were also concerned about the hair mattresses, which were 'too thin'. As a remedy, they recommended that an upholstery shop should be opened.[40] By 1872 the bedding was recorded as being 'good, sufficient and quite clean'. Straw mattresses, however, were still in use: 38 on the male side and 28 on the female side.[41] As the asylum became more crowded, the bedding situation worsened: straw mattresses continued to be used and in some wards patients slept on the floor or had to crawl over other patients' beds to get to their own.

Sanitation in the Victorian asylum was usually basic and was a constant source of comment and concern for the Commissioners and Visitors. The standard of hygiene was judged partly by sight but also by the presence or absence of 'smells'. The Visitors made frequent references to cleanliness and odours in their reports, claiming for example that everything was in excellent order and 'there was no offensive smell whatever, even in the idiots' ward on either side'[42] or that:

> The wards were all clean and in good order as were the dormitories nor was there any bad smell or want of ventilation except slight effluvia in the dormitory of No 6 ward. On the male side there was no patient either in seclusion or shut in his room and the dormitories and wards were perfectly clean and free from any effusive smell whatever.[43]

There was always a great shortage of toilets in the asylum. A Visitor in March 1864 noted that 'The new water closet is finished for No 6 ward and is a great convenience: a similar one is required for several other wards as some of them have only one seat for 90 patients.'[44] The shortage of toilets was matched by a lack of washbasins in the dormitories. Denne had advised the Visitors soon after the asylum opened that he wanted to have some stands for washbasins in the larger dormitories. Ventilation was also a cause for concern in the first few months of opening. Visitors repeatedly remarked on the lack of ventilation and Denne proposed to remedy it by installing ventilators in the floors and having the windows kept open as much as possible.

There were frequent water shortages due to the inadequate underground supply discovered during the original building works. This meant that patients had to share bath water. The Commissioners strongly disapproved of the practice and monitored the situation closely on their yearly visits. By 1867 the water problems had not been solved and the Commissioners registered their disappointment that there had not been the 'desired amendment', as up to four patients continued to be bathed in the same water.[45] Two years later the situation had still not improved and the Commissioners reported that 'no good excuse seems to exist why, in future, each patient should not have clean water'.

While the new asylum seemed to provide substantially better living conditions than the old Bedford Asylum, it is difficult to gauge any definite reactions. Neither patients nor staff recorded their initial impressions of their new surroundings, and all that remains are a few short comments which found their way into the official record.

Gender and Architecture

The organisation of the Victorian asylum was based on the separation of the sexes. This social division was reflected architecturally, as all asylums were designed to include separate male and female wings with separate staff. The segregation of the sexes was an enduring legacy of the Victorian asylum, and in most mental hospitals this division remained in existence until the 1960s. Victorian norms of extreme modesty and decorum, as well as fear of sexual contact, ensured that rules of segregation were strictly enforced. Male doctors could only speak to a female patient if she was chaperoned by the matron. At Bedford Asylum, Denne had been criticised by the Commissioners for allowing male patients to carry out some of the heavier jobs in the laundry. The segregation of patients was extended to include staff. A rule book dated 1876 states clearly that:

> no Male Attendant, Servant, or Patient shall be allowed to enter the female wards, or any female to enter the male wards, except in cases where the Resident Medical Superintendent shall deem it advisable.[46]

The security arrangements of asylums were carefully checked by the Commissioners.[47] Despite these precautions, however, unmarried female patients did occasionally become pregnant. When this happened, vigorous attempts were made to establish paternity and both male patients and staff members came under scrutiny. The usual procedure following a birth was for the baby to be handed over to the Guardians of the mother's home parish or, if the mother was a vagrant, the child would be sent to the local workhouse.[48]

It is not known whether the first group of twelve patients who transferred from Bedford travelled in the same train but, if they did, they separated on arrival. The six women and the female attendants entered the new building through the female entrance, and the six males and male attendants entered through the male entrance. From then onwards, the two groups would only be in each other's company in certain strictly controlled social situations, such as occasional supervised recreational events and in the chapel. The guidelines for the design of asylum chapels stated explicitly that the sexes, although they were to enter the chapel separately, could worship together. In front of

God, patients shared a common humanity which did not translate into the realm of daily social life.

While all patients were under surveillance, or 'careful watching' as it was called by the Victorians, women were more carefully watched than men.[49] There were some protections in place for patients – they could speak to the Visiting Committee members for example. There was also an advocates group who called themselves 'The Alleged Lunatics' Friend Society'. It was founded by Richard Paternoster and John Perceval in 1845 and had as its stated intention 'the protection of the British subject from unjust confinement on the grounds of mental derangement'. The group were very active in raising funds and would obtain legal advice and even fight cases where they thought someone had been improperly detained. When the Alleged Lunatics' Friend Society protested at the censorship of patients' mail, their category of 'patient' excluded women. Women, they agreed, needed to be protected against the possibility of indecorous self-revelation.[50]

Women were admitted to asylums in larger numbers and appear to have had longer periods of hospitalisation. They also had lower death rates than male patients. The reasons for women outnumbering men are complex, but are likely related to poverty, social circumstances and the greater difficulty impoverished and abandoned women encountered in being granted subsistence payments.[51]

Female patients often surprised the staff and visiting dignitaries with their rowdiness, obscene language and 'excitement'. In the Victorian context such behaviour from women was scandalous and the male asylum doctors struggled to explain it. Their answers were usually based on ideas of female biology and its inherent weaknesses. One explanation suggested that control in the female mind is solely dependent on religious and moral principles. When the mind is weakened by insanity, women are prone to becoming obscene and rowdy.[52] Alternative explanations, such as the fact that women had fewer opportunities than men to move within the asylum building, to take part in active recreation or to participate in outdoor activity, seem rarely to have been considered. It was believed that the solution to women's rowdiness was industrious work designed to allow them little time to talk.

Entertainment

Various supervised forms of entertainment and amusement were integral to asylum life for both patients and staff where segregation still operated but less strictly. In 1861 Denne reported that:

> entertainments were held every fortnight, in the evening, dancing, etc ... also the band, formed by the attendants, forms a praiseworthy part of their duty for the patients' comfort: and at the Christmas

parties an addition was made to the supper of sandwiches, cake etc
... a representation of the 'Ethiopian Serenaders' was got up by the
attendants.[53]

The staff often held their own entertainments as well. A particularly
rowdy one in July 1861 was brought to the attention of the Visiting
Committee, who called for an inquiry. The report stated that 89 people
were present at the entertainment, including attendants and their wives,
artisans, farm labourers and a few people unconnected with the asylum.
The festivities began at 8pm and lasted until 6am the next morning.
Dancing was going on the whole time in the three day rooms on
the male side of the asylum, the doors being left open so they joined
together to make one large area. The steward reported that 36 bottles
of wine and spirits were taken from the medical stores and Denne, who
stayed until 5am, had supervised their distribution. Approximately 160
quarts of beer and porter were also distributed to anyone who asked
for them. This, the Committee noted, came to two quarts of beer and
porter and a half pint of spirits for every person present, the removal of
which had nowhere been recorded in the issue books.

The farm bailiff, who had not attended the party, reported to
the Committee that on his way to work at 6am he saw one of the
attendant's wives being led home by two other women, all of whom
seemed to be 'in a state of intoxication'. He found the cowman lying in
a state of unconscious drunkenness by the road near the farm buildings
and a young man employed in the same department lying near him in
a similar condition. The farm labourers did not report to work until
10am in the morning, and those who arrived earlier to help with the
milking 'were not in a fit state to do it'. The Committee resolved to
'express a strong condemnation of the want of efficient supervision and
care shown in this case by the medical superintendent and to admonish
him to a more cautious conduct of these entertainments in future'.[54]

By 1863, in addition to the usual entertainments at Midsummer
and Christmas, and the fortnightly dances, the Committee of Visitors
agreed that amateur theatricals could be started. During the winter
evenings, scenery was made and the shows produced for an audience
of selected patients, members of the Visiting Committee and other
local dignitaries. This began a long tradition of amateur theatre which
became associated with the asylum. Other forms of recreation included
large walking parties. Accompanied by attendants, these large groups of
patients took long walks into the countryside, primarily on Sundays.

By 1869 other forms of entertainment had been added, including
monthly readings at which, according to the annual report, Denne, the
Rev. Butt and members of their families assisted, as well as some of their

friends who lived in the neighbourhood. The library had expanded and consisted of 3796 books.

An essential aspect of an asylum was its cricket ground. At TCA the cricket ground was laid out during 1862 and 1863. The medical superintendent noted that cricket proved a great source of healthy recreation in the summer evenings, many of the patients being able to watch the game although they were not included in the teams that played. Male patients thronged the airing courts which looked out onto the cricket field, their faces pressed against the wrought-iron rails. This relegation of patients to an onlooker role raises an interesting issue in recreation and entertainment in the Victorian asylum. While there was much emphasis on the importance of entertainment, which was seen to be therapeutic for patients, organised programmes appear to have primarily encouraged patients to play a passive role. Although patients danced and walked, they did not play cricket, nor become members of the choir, band or theatre. Rather, they were entertained by the attendants who took the lead and played the active roles. Thus, while recreational activities were believed to be therapeutic, they were therapeutic only from the perspective of passive involvement.[55]

Patients were allowed to have visitors on Mondays, Tuesdays, Wednesdays and Saturdays between 10am and 4pm and at all times in the case of dangerous illness. Visits, however, could be restricted if the medical superintendent thought that they might be injurious to the patient concerned. Patients were permitted to have private conversations with their friends and could make complaints. Visitors of the opposite sex, however, could not remain in a room with a patient unless an attendant or third person was present.[56]

The Commissioners in Lunacy

Most of what we know about TCA in its early days is based on the asylum's official reports and records, including the Visitors' monthly reports, the annual reports and the minutes of the various committees. The yearly reports of the Commissioners in Lunacy give detailed accounts of the running of the institution, general impressions of the asylum and suggestions for improvements. They provide useful glimpses into the day-to-day problems, deficiencies and realities of life in the asylum.

The Commissioners made their first visit to TCA shortly after it was opened in April 1860. In general they were favourably impressed with what they found. While they acknowledged that much still needed to be done, they praised the Committee of Visitors, the superintendent and the matron for 'the zeal and activity they display in its management'.[57] Much of their report is concerned with practical matters: the numbers of patients in the asylum, the number of deaths since the opening, patients' behaviour and the size of the congregation at chapel on Sundays. Food was a tangible category which the Commissioners could use to evaluate the quality of care in the asylum. In their first report, the Commissioners stated that they 'saw the patients at dinner and tasted the food, consisting of meat and potato pies, which were very good and well cooked'. They noted that while beer was not allowed at dinner, it was given to the working patients at luncheon. Half a pint of beer was given to each patient on Sundays. They failed to note, though, that those who worked got more food, and that men always got more than women. Neither did they describe the mealtime routine in the segregated dining halls, which involved the tedious counting and recounting of every item of cutlery.

The first report made a series of recommendations which 'require the earliest attention':

> The airing courts should be levelled without delay as they at present are unsafe for feeble and paralytic patients.
>
> The number of chairs and comfortable seats with backs should be greatly increased, especially in the wards used for epileptic and feeble patients.
>
> A stock of books and periodicals is much required and generally the means of amusement should be increased.

Airing courts, large outdoor areas surrounded by high railings, were a standard feature of asylum architecture. Patients who could not be employed in the various departments of the asylum spent long hours in the airing courts. A 1908 article in a Cambridge newspaper provides a description of the airing courts at Fulbourn Asylum:

> In both wings large walled-in exercise yards, officially termed 'airing courts', adjoin the day rooms, with broad asphalt paths and grass plots ... One of the first things to rivet my attention on visiting the exercise yard was a long string of men and youths, hand in hand, walking ponderously and in a pitiful aimless fashion, backwards and forwards along one of the paths. It was only by such companionship, I was assured, that these patients could be induced to take any exercise at all. Left to themselves, they would prop their persons against the walls. It was very pitiable to see so many young people amongst the patients.[58]

In 1861 the Commissioners reported for the year that 129 patients had been admitted, 44 discharged and 47 had died (see table below). Of the

460 patients in the asylum, 212 were men and 248 women, four of whom were out on leave. The Commissioners reported that the patients were generally 'quiet and orderly and clean, and properly clothed. The wards were clean and well ventilated.'[59] When they enquired about patient occupations, amusements and attendance at chapel they were advised that:

> on average 125 men and 131 women are regularly employed. Of the men 66 work in the garden and farm and 21 are occupied in workshops as smiths, shoemakers, tailors, carpenters, painters etc. Thirty-three of the women work regularly in the laundry and wash house and the rest assist in the ward, and work at their needle. The attendance at chapel averages 115 men and 71 women.[60]

The report concludes that the new asylum is not quite up to standard, and that 'although great progress has been made and much has been done to improve the general condition of the institution, much still remains to be effected before it can be considered as in a thoroughly efficient state'.[61] As for the previous year's recommendations, some progress had been made in levelling the airing courts, but they still required turfing, planting and gravelling; some of the requested furniture had been supplied with more on order; and a small stock of books had been procured. They also recommended that rules be drawn up to regulate the duties of the steward, assistant clerk and storekeeper, assistant matron, nurses and attendants, and that every ward should be supplied more completely with conveniences such as proper fittings in the sculleries, looking glasses, washstands and seats in the bedrooms.[62]

The report closes with concerns about the accounts, which were 'very irregularly kept'. The cost of maintaining a patient in the asylum had risen from 9/- to 10/- per week and the Commissioners worried that this increase would 'no doubt have an influence in reference to the early transmission of patients to the asylum'. To remedy this, they suggested that perhaps some of the staff might have their wages reduced. Not surprisingly this proved to be a very unpopular suggestion which was not taken up.

By 1862, the number of patients had increased to 485. During the previous year, 129 new patients had been admitted. Forty-four patients had recovered and been discharged; 47 had died – all from 'ordinary causes'. During their visit, the Commissioners saw two newly admitted patients who were 'decidedly insane'. They remarked that the sanitary condition of the asylum was good, and since the opening of the asylum there had been no epidemics. Denne advised the Commissioners that 'the general condition and habits of the patients of the worst class removed to the asylum from Bedford has been materially improved by

Year	Admissions			Recovered			Deaths			Total Dec. 31		
	M	F	T	M	F	T	M	F	T	M	F	T
1860	225	269	494	9	22	31	27	11	38	186	237	423
1861	59	70	129	10	34	44	23	24	47	212	248	460
1862	73	71	144	23	29	52	29	27	56	227	258	485
1863	63	58	121	24	28	52	28	15	43	237	266	503
1864	56	64	120	28	23	51	35	29	64	229	276	505
1865	66	82	148	27	37	64	26	33	59	242	286	528
1866	59	75	134	24	31	55	28	46	74	242	277	519
1867	69	74	143	34	30	64	34	24	58	243	265	508
1868	65	73	138	25	34	59	24	30	54	242	263	505
1869	65	83	148	20	37	57	29	41	70	248	261	509
1870	81	84	165	13	35	48	44	36	80	265	268	533

Admissions, Recovery Rates and Deaths 1860–70 [63]

the change'. 297 patients were employed and the chapel attendance the previous day was 195. On visiting the wards they noted that, 'With a few exceptions in the lower female ward we found the patients tranquil and orderly, their personal condition as to clothing and otherwise reflected credit on the attendants.'[64] Interestingly, they praised the staff for using an atypical approach to patients who were disturbed and destructive:

> We are glad to record that no special dresses are provided as in most other asylums, for patients of destructive propensities, such patients are supplied with old clothes which they may tear up if they please. At the same time they are allowed extra bread throughout the day and also in some cases at night. The results of the treatment adopted is stated to be a speedy cessation of the habit.[65]

The remainder of the report refers to improvements that have been made in painting and decorating on the male side, and additions of furniture and books. In one of the first references to the increasing number of patients, especially women, the Commissioners noted that one of the male dormitories was to be turned into a female ward. They commended the Dennes for their successful management of the asylum and attention to the care and comfort of patients. The Commissioners were also shown the seclusion records and noted that while seclusion was used in most instances for very short times, women were more likely to be secluded than men, and that three quarters of the patients secluded were epileptic. In their report of 1867 the Commissioners recorded that, since their last visit, 37 men had been secluded on 506 separate occasions, and 42 women had been secluded on 129 occasions. The Commissioners were, however, doubtful that every instance was noted and the real numbers were probably higher than the official record stated.

Madness and Epilepsy

In the 1860s there was no effective medication to control epilepsy. Initially epileptic patients at TCA were cared for in dormitories alongside other patients. In 1872 the Commissioners noted that an epileptic patient had recently died of asphyxia and suggested that, as in other asylums, special wards in each division be provided for epileptic and suicidal patients. They also suggested that a special night attendant be employed who had no other duties.

Each month the Committee of Visitors' monthly report recorded the number of patients ill in bed. Inevitably this number included patients who were having seizures or recovering from seizures. William Lynn Smart, a Visitor in June 1860, noted that there were seven females in bed (four from mania and three from epilepsy), and seven males (one from paralysis, one from debility and five from epilepsy).[66] In April 1861 it was noted that there were seven females in their cells, four from epilepsy and three from paralysis, with three of the epileptic patients in an excited state.[67] The following month's Visitor described the chief forms of suffering in the asylum to be 'epilepsy, paralysis, and debility'.[68]

Seizures were not only frequent but often violent and lengthy. Patients who were having seizures were sometimes placed in padded rooms to protect them from physical injury. The Visitors' report of March 1864 noted that 'Three females were in the padded rooms but not on account of their being violent but because the acute fits of epilepsy were on them.'[69] Physical injury during seizures was common. The Visitors' report of 17 July 1860 stated that M.B. had broken her arm by falling down when in a fit.

A typical case history of an epileptic patient was that of F.L. who was admitted to TCA in April 1863. He was an unmarried 21-year-old whose father was a labourer. The admission notes described him as 'rather stout, 5 feet 3 in height – well nourished – head rather large – eyes blind – skin healthy'. F.L. had 'been insane for about 3 years and is also an epileptic. [He] was previously under treatment at the Union Workhouse but has lately become violent and dangerous to others. He becomes much worse when he has an epileptic fit. At other times he is quiet.' By July 1863 it was noted that he had had one rather violent episode since entering the asylum which precipitated his being kept in his room for a few days. His condition was otherwise unchanged.[70] A month later he had had attacks of excitement which caused him to be confined in his room again, at which times he became 'very dirty in his habits and noisy'.[71] In October he continued 'fat and in good condition. Still has fits of excitement at times when the epileptic fits come on.'[72] By January of 1864 his health was about the same but the epileptic fits and fits of excitement were less frequent. Four months later on, the notes recorded that his epileptic attacks occurred about every month or six weeks, 'when he becomes very noisy and dirty'.

For the next three years his condition was recorded as unchanged. In 1869 he continued 'to have frequent fits, at such times is obstinate and violent, is quite blind. Health good.'[73] F.L.'s final case note on 12 June 1876 merely stated that he 'has had more frequent fits of late: two days ago he had a succession, the lungs became congested and he died today from exhaustion after epilepsy'.[74]

The Working Life of the Asylum

The nineteenth-century asylum was a place where both staff and inmates worked. Social and economic factors combined to ensure that work was a central aspect of patient life. Victorian lunacy reformers had strong ideas about the therapeutic value of work for the mentally ill. It was believed that if patients were working they would forget about their illnesses, which in turn would help them to recover. The number of patients in 'gainful employment' was a frequent category for comment in official reports. The first Annual Report notes that:

> the patients are now employed as much as possible under the inspection of the attendants and it is a very gratifying sight to see numbers of men working happily on different parts of the farm forgetful for a time of their unhappy condition ... [B]esides those who work on the farm a considerable number of the patients are daily employed in the laundries and workshops and the remainder whose imbecility renders them incapable of work are amused in either the day rooms or large airing courts.[75]

There was another less-commented-upon aspect of patient employment. Patients worked to sustain the asylum community. Without patient labour the sheer scale of the institutional system would have been unworkable. As Valentine, writing about the Horton Asylum, explains:

> The economy of the asylum depended on patient labour. They worked, if they were capable of it, because work was supposed to be good for them. But they also worked because the asylum system, farm, laundry, kitchen, shoemakers and all, would collapse without them.[76]

The economic importance of patient labour at Three Counties Asylum was highlighted by Marlborough Pryor, first Chairman of the Committee of Visitors, when he claimed that the Committee were looking forward with confidence to the time when the profits of the farm would enable them to reduce the costs of maintenance. As the patients became more productive it became cheaper to house and feed them. By 1864, Pryor's predictions were realised as the farm results were 'highly satisfactory', enabling the rates to be dropped to 8/– a week.

While the authorities extolled the value of patient work, we do not know what the patients themselves thought about this compulsory aspect of asylum life. Interviews with people who were patients in the 1950s, just prior to the banning of patient labour as exploitative, suggest that for some work was an important and meaningful aspect of their lives, while for others it was drudgery. In neither case – the nineteenth-century decision that patients should work, or the twentieth-century decision that they should not – did patients have any input or choice.

Patients worked in all departments of the asylum. In December 1864 there were 229 male and 276 female patients in the institution. Of these, 130 men and 180 women were employed. These numbers included 60 men who worked on the land, six who worked as shoemakers, three who worked as tailors, four as carpenters and two as painters (the remainder were deemed unskilled and carried out the many menial tasks required around the asylum such as sweeping and cleaning). Of the women, 42 worked in the laundry and the remainder were employed in sewing, straw work, in the kitchen or helping on the wards. While the annual reports proudly emphasised the number of patients working, we are told little of how the remaining 194 patients spent their time. Undoubtedly some of them were incapacitated or elderly and infirm. Frequent complaints were made by hospital administrators that they were sent a considerable number of patients suffering from senile dementia rather than mental illness. These numbers, however, would have only accounted for a proportion of the unemployed patients. As work was not adapted to patients' abilities but, rather, patients had to adapt to the jobs available, those who could not carry out the assigned tasks remained unemployed. The reality was that in the large Victorian asylums significant numbers of patients had nothing to do and simply sat day after day on the wards or out in the airing courts.

Where possible, patients were employed at their previous occupations. One of the first patients admitted to TCA, J.K., a 38-year-old cabinet maker, was employed from his admission in 1860 until shortly before his death in 1877 in the carpenter's shop. His medical notes revolve largely around his continuation of his trade in the asylum. In 1865 he is reported to be 'about the same since he has been here – is very incoherent but quiet and does a great deal of work at his trade'. A few random notes over the next ten years mostly reiterate that he continued to work in the carpenter's shop and that his condition was unchanged. Some time later he was reported to be in good health but 'full of delusions', apparently believing himself to be a Sir Henry Bland.

His penultimate entry noted that he 'should do no work' and the final entry on 31 December 1877 merely states 'died', with no cause of death recorded.[77]

Laundry work was believed to be particularly beneficial for women. Valentine suggests that this was 'presumably because it provided some kind of physical exercise'.[78] In 1864, 42 women were employed in the laundry, one of whom was K.B. (see p. 33). The majority of the entries in her sparse medical notes refer firstly to the fact that she worked in the laundry and only secondly to her mental state. K.B.'s existence is therefore almost entirely defined by the fact that she was a laundry worker. Yet we have no idea of her daily experience of work. The official record merely informs us that in 1888 a new day room was added to the laundry, and in 1898 it was decided to enlarge and improve the laundry at a cost of £1,350. Visitors frequently complained that the floor of the laundry was too wet. There is little that we can deduce from this information to help us understand K.B.'s experiences of her daily work other than the fact that the wet floor was probably dangerous and that the working conditions at times were probably cramped and arduous.

The only descriptions we have of patient work come from the official record. The Visitor of the month for February 1886 writes in his report that on his way to the asylum he met two large parties of patients going to work. He noted that they appeared 'very quiet but bright and cheerful'. The same report observed that a female patient got her hand caught in a machine in the laundry (perhaps a mangle). We are told nothing of how the accident happened nor details of the patient's injury. We are simply told that 'all is going on satisfactorily'.

The asylum's daily routine revolved around work. Unfortunately no records outlining the daily routine at the Three Counties Asylum survive. The routine, however, is likely to have been similar to that reported for the Horton Asylum by Valentine.[79]

Daily Routine

Breakfast	8.30am
Start work	9–9.30am
Lunch (a snack)	10–10.30am
Back to ward	12.00
Dinner	12.30pm
Back to work	2–2.30pm
Back to ward	4.30pm
Tea	5.00pm

In 1906 a new medical superintendent took over at Horton and was appalled at what he considered the laxity of the asylum's work habits.

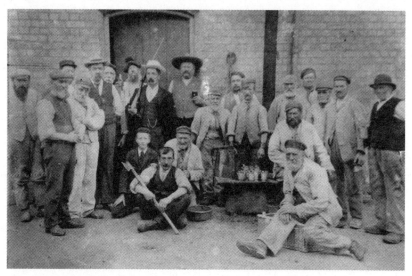

Figure 2.3 *Asylum farm labourers, c.1890*

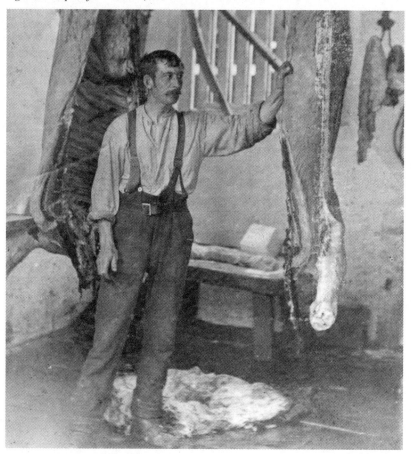

Figure 2.4 *The Butcher's shop, c.1890*

Accordingly he drew up a new work routine which enabled him to 'get two-and-a-half hours per day more work from each working patient'. Fortunately there are no reports of similar happenings at TCA.

The 1845 Lunacy Act ensured that the mentally ill in each county had access to what was considered to be the cutting edge of care – an asylum in the country. Regulated carefully and inspected yearly by the Commissioners in Lunacy, the county asylums were an improvement on the previous often brutal regime of private unregulated asylums. Situated in rural settings, the asylums were surrounded by attractive grounds which provided those who were acutely ill with a place of refuge in which to recover. The spectacular landscape, however, was matched by an unspectacular range of treatments. For many who entered an asylum in the nineteenth century the supposed brief admission to a refuge in the country often became a lifetime in a rural backwater. The all-encompassing institution provided for every supposed need, and those that could not be met were eventually forgotten, as patients, and also staff, settled into an orderly but little-changing routine. The long asylum era had just begun and it was to be ninety years before its place as the ultimate in care for the mentally ill was seriously challenged.

Notes

1   A. Scull, *Museums of Madness: The Social Organisation of Insanity in Nineteenth Century England.* Allen Lane 1979, 208.
2   *Ibid.*, 209.
3   Commissioners in Lunacy, 2nd Annual Report 1847, quoted in Scull 1979, 210.
4   LT5/6 Annual Reports of the Visiting Committee, 1860.
5   LT6/6, General Rules and Regulations and Orders for the Government of the Lunatic Asylum for the Counties of Bedford, Hertford and Huntingdon, 1878.
6   M. Stevens, *Life in the Victorian Asylum*, Pen & Sword Books, Barnsley 2014, 96–7.
7   LT5/6, 1878.
8   LT5/6, 1860.
9   B. Cashman, *A Proper House: Bedford Lunatic Asylum 1812–1860.* North Bedfordshire Health Authority 1992, 138.
10   *Cambridge Chronicle*, 6 Nov 1858.
11   LT5/6, 1860.
12   Admissions Register, 1860.
13   LF29, Female Case Books, 1864, 1875, 1886; LF46, Burial Register, 1889.
14   Admissions Register, 1860.
15   *Ibid.*, LF46, 1897.
16   Admissions Register, 1860; LF46, 1889.
17   Chaplain's Journal, 14 July 1859.
18   LF4/6/1, Building Sub-committee Minutes, 20 Sept 1858.
19   LF4/6/1, 20 Nov 1858.
20   Cashman 1992, 153.
21   LT6/6, Rules and Regulations.
22   *Ibid.*

23   *Ibid.*
24   For more information on S. Wing, see Cashman 1992, 111, 113–17.
25   LF1/1, Oct 1859.
26   LF1/1, Feb 1861.
27   LF1/1, Mar 1861.
28   *Ibid.*
29   Quoted in Cashman 1992, 138.
30   Noted in Cashman 1992, 138.
31   LT5/6, 1860.
32   J. Taylor, *Hospital and Asylum Architecture in England 1840–1914: Building for Health Care.* Mansell Publishing 1991, 166.
33   Quoted in Taylor 1991, 166.
34   *Ibid.*
35   Nicholas Bridges, personal communication June 1998.
36   LF4/1/1a, Committee of Visitors Minutes of Visit, 7 May 1860.
37   LF4/5, 1860.
38   *Ibid.*
39   *Ibid.*
40   *Ibid.*, 1868.
41   *Ibid.*, 1872.
42   LF4/1/1a, 30 Apr 1861.
43   *Ibid.*, 4 Apr 1861.
44   *Ibid.*, 4 Mar 1864.
45   *Ibid.*, 18 Dec 1867.
46   LT6/6, 1878.
47   In their Annual Report of 1871 the Commissioners objected to the mixing of the sexes in the mortuary at Fulbourn Asylum in Cambridgeshire (quoted in A. Scull, *Social Order/Mental Disorder: Anglo-American Psychiatry in Historical Perspective.* University of California Press 1989, 273).
48   E. Showalter, 'Victorian Women and Insanity' in A. Scull (ed.) *Madhouses, Mad-Doctors, and Madmen: The Social History of Psychiatry in the Victorian Era.* Athlone Press 1981, 320.
49   *Ibid.*, 319.
50   *Ibid.*
51   *Ibid.*, 316–18.
52   J. Bucknill, *Manual of Psychological Medicine* 1871, 273 quoted in Showalter 1981, 320.
53   LF4/5. 1861
54   LF1/1, 22 Jul 1861.
55   This is in direct contrast to the contemporary emphasis in Occupational Therapy, Drama Therapy and Art Therapy which stresses the therapeutic importance of participation.
56   LT6/6, 1878.
57   LF4/5, 1860.
58   Quoted in Clark 1996, 19.
59   LF4/5, 1861.
60   *Ibid.*
61   *Ibid.*
62   *Ibid.*
63   LF3/4, Asylum Reports, 1860–90.
64   LF4/5, 1862.
65   *Ibid.*

66   LF4/1/1a, 14 June 1860.
67   *Ibid.*, 4 Apr 1861.
68   *Ibid.*, 20 May 1861.
69   *Ibid.*, 4 Mar 1864.
70   Patient case notes.
71   *Ibid.*
72   *Ibid.*
73   *Ibid.*
74   *Ibid.*
75   LT5/6 Annual Reports of the Visiting Committee, 1860.
76   R. Valentine, *Asylum Hospital, Haven: A History of Horton Hospital.* Riverside
     Mental Health Trust 1996, 35–6.
77   Patient case notes.
78   Valentine 1996, 38.
79   *Ibid.*, 35.

CHAPTER THREE

Edwardian Psychiatry
and the First World War

A sylum life changed little in the decades between the opening of TCA and the turn of the twentieth century. Patients were still expected to gain the greatest benefit from exposure to a regimented life, industrious work and fresh country air.

The twentieth century, however, was to witness dramatic changes with the introduction of an array of radical new therapies and an active medical/scientific approach to treatment. The effect of these changes slowly began to appear at TCA following the massive upheavals in British society resulting from the First World War.

Outwardly the war seemed to have little effect on the day-to-day life of the asylum, but it did usher in some significant changes. A number of male staff enlisted at the outset of the war, but an exemption from active service was obtained for asylum attendants and few went after the initial recruitment. The main concession to the war effort, particularly after rationing was introduced, was an increased attempt at self-sufficiency in food production. One of the biggest changes the asylum saw between 1910 and 1920 was the admission of two new classes of patients: shell-shocked soldiers and the criminally insane. The

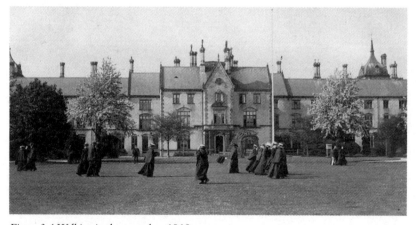

Figure 3.1 Walking in the grounds, c. 1910

first criminal cases were taken in 1911 and the asylum began admitting discharged soldiers suffering from shell-shock in 1917. The first decades of the new century also saw a number of changes to the working conditions of asylum staff, including the recognition of a union and a superannuation act. Life within the asylum not only reflected these changes, but was also punctuated by a series of noteworthy events, including outbreaks of diseases, the death of the asylum brewer in a vat of beer, the building of a pathology laboratory and the conversion of the isolation hospital to a ward for private patients.

Private Patients Scheme

A separate section of the asylum to be set aside for private patients had been talked about as early as 1896.[1] Nothing was done about it until over a decade later, although a handful of patients classed as private had been housed with the general patient population since the 1890s. In the intervening years, the distinction between paupers and private patients was less clear. This was highlighted by the case of two sisters from Hitchin, admitted to the asylum in 1909. On admission they were found to have large sums of money on them totalling nearly £300. This was an amount equivalent to the annual salary of the asylum chaplain. The money was paid to the treasurer of their parish union for safekeeping and the local Clerk of the Board of Guardians inquired of the Visiting Committee whether or not the sisters should be transferred to the private class. The Committee had never been asked to judge whether a patient should be admitted as a pauper or private patient before and there was no allowance for making such a judgement in the 1890 Lunacy Act. Section 3 of the Act simply stated that a patient could be classified as private if the patient had the financial means. At TCA the difference between a private and pauper patient had been in name only and 'merely a matter of sentiment', both receiving the same treatment. If a patient's family could afford to pay the maintenance fee, the patient could be classified as a private patient and thus the stigma of being labelled a pauper would not be added to that of mental illness.

The Committee decided to leave the decision in this case to the local Board of Guardians. The incident was important in another sense because, in the course of their inquiries, the Committee found that other county asylums were setting aside special accommodation for private patients 'just above the pauper class' where better treatment could be had for increased rates. This stimulated their interest in providing the same kind of service for a small profit.[2] They began contacting other asylums to see how the scheme worked.

An initial plan was proposed in early 1911 to convert the existing isolation hospital, which was being used to treat female tuberculosis cases, to a separate facility for 25 private patients by the addition of single rooms and a conservatory. A veranda to accommodate the tuberculosis patients would be built off the infirmary of the main building. Private patients in the main building would continue to be charged at £1 per week while private patients in the separate hospital would be charged at 30/- per week plus 5/- if a separate room was provided. Patients would be allowed to wear their own clothes and in the private rooms might have some of their own furniture.[3]

The conversion of the isolation hospital for private care required making suitable arrangements for a replacement isolation facility. Wilbury Farm, which bordered on the asylum property, had been leased by the asylum from Trinity College, Cambridge for a number of years and the Visiting Committee were interested in using the farm buildings as additional accommodation for 'quiet' patients or possibly as a substitute for the isolation hospital. However, the water supply to the farm was not sufficient to meet the needs of multiple residents. The cost of linking the water lines from the main supply to the farm would be high and Trinity College refused to pay. The Committee were not keen on making such a large investment in property not owned by the asylum and eventually negotiated the purchase of the farm in 1911 for £5000.

The Lunacy Commission gave their approval in late 1911 for the conversion of the isolation hospital to a private patients' facility, subject to another building being constructed in advance of the conversion for use as an isolation unit. It was decided to adapt Wilbury Farm for the purpose.[4] Soon after this decision was made the Visiting Committee were advised that new regulations for separate housing of mental defectives were soon to be passed. Under the provisions of the Mental Deficiency Act 1913, counties were to provide separate accommodation for the mentally deficient (i.e. people with learning disabilities) as opposed to the mentally ill. This had been proposed at TCA as early as 1894 when a Visitor remarked that he was struck by the number of 'idiots mixed up together with the ordinary inmates. A separate classification and a separate building for idiots seems eminently desirable.'[5] It was decided to leave the question of the isolation hospital until it was determined whether or not Wilbury Farm would be required to house mental defectives. This, in effect, meant that the scheme for private patients had to be postponed as well. With the onset of the war, the scheme was further postponed and was not taken up again until the war ended (see p. 68).

Typhoid, Tuberculosis and Smallpox

The isolation hospital, though not in constant use, was periodically required to house patients during outbreaks of infectious diseases. Any such outbreak was viewed with alarm since so many patients lived in such close quarters. During the 1902 smallpox outbreak all patients in the asylum were vaccinated and the asylum was closed to visitors for seven months. It was made mandatory that all 'lunatic tramps' have their clothing destroyed on admission, as the clothes were considered a possible source of disease transmission. The Guardians of the local unions were to pay for supplying new clothing if the inmate left the institution.[6] In 1903 there was another minor outbreak of smallpox and the asylum was closed again for a month.

Tuberculosis was a constant threat and there was a fairly high annual death rate among patients. It was decided in 1906 to look at the question of providing additional isolated accommodation for tubercular patients. The committee recommended that verandas be built on the outside of the female and male ground-floor dormitories and the isolation hospital to accommodate the new open-air treatment being recommended for tuberculosis. Samuel de Lisle, who had succeeded Swain as medical superintendent in 1906, was authorised by the Visiting Committee to visit asylums which had begun using the open-air treatment to determine the costs, results of treatment and the best form for constructing verandas. The results must have been positive since on hearing de Lisle's report the Visiting Committee recommended that plans and estimates be commissioned for verandas which were to have glass roofs that were colour-washed in summer and clear in winter.[7]

Tuberculosis was regarded as a routine though serious illness and a certain number of cases were expected as a matter of course. Smallpox, though seen as very grave, was only an occasional threat. Outbreaks of dysentery, however, were quite common and there were often deaths associated with them. For example, in the summer of 1911 there was an unusually serious outbreak of 'summer diarrhoea' and a number of the elderly patients died as a result.

The most feared disease and a constant hazard due to the asylum water-supply problems was typhoid. An outbreak in 1906 was particularly threatening to the asylum as it drew the Visiting Committee into an expensive lawsuit. In September, the farm bailiff, Mr Brown, reported ill with typhoid fever. The water supply was checked and though it was not particularly good in some respects it was not considered to contain typhoid pathogens. Soon after, however, five male patients were also found to have milder cases of typhoid and were isolated. A nurse from outside was hired by the Visiting Committee to tend to the bailiff, who by then was seriously ill. Mr Brown died on 1 October and the next day a special meeting of the Visiting Committee was convened to assess the situation.

In 1875–6 there had been problems with sewage leaking into the water supply and work had been done to prevent it from getting in again by blocking up the sources. An examination of the original blocked sites by the asylum engineer showed some small leaks at the repair site and in the walls of the well. The water samples examined when the bailiff first fell ill had not been taken from these sites, and it was agreed that samples be taken at the leakage points and sent for bacteriological analysis.[8] The results of this test were not recorded in the official minutes of the Visiting Committee. The only reference to the test was an approval to pay the bacteriologist, Sir Thomas Stevenson, of Guy's Hospital, for his analyses. However, in subsequent references to the water problems·the situation was always referred to as the 'pollution of wells'.

A London firm was asked to supply an estimate for a waterproof lining for the wells, and on visiting the site the cost was estimated at between £3000 and £4000. In the meantime it was recommended to the medical superintendent that all drinking water be filtered, an option not considered practical on a hospital–wide basis, though two filters were fitted, one in the surgery and one in the aeration plant. The Committee began looking for an alternative to relining the wells as the expense was considered far too great.

By the middle of October there had been eighteen cases of typhoid and five patients had died.[9] In November, the Visiting Committee received a letter from the bailiff's widow asking for financial help, preferably a pension for her husband's service, as she was in very difficult circumstances. The Committee reported that they could not grant her any pension. The best they could do was give her £10 from the asylum hardship fund. At this point the drainage system of the asylum was examined, particularly those drains close to the wells. The whole system was found to be in a defective state, with some lavatory drains leaking at a number of places, and the laundry drains leaking at all joints. The Visiting Committee immediately postponed the repairs to the wells until the drainage system had been thoroughly inspected and repaired, with all drains in the vicinity of the wells replaced with iron piping. Soon after this resolution another case of typhoid appeared and it was agreed that it was probably linked to the same outbreak. Once the drainage repairs were completed, it was decided to use the asylum bricklayers to cement the interior lining of the wells, closing one well at a time to allow the work to be done and thereby avoiding the high cost of the plan tendered by the outside firm.

In March 1907, the Visiting Committee received a letter from the solicitors of the bailiff's widow asking for £1000 compensation for the loss of her husband. The Committee resolved to deny all liability and defend any action, should they receive a writ. By June the action had been started. Brown's widow claimed that her husband died from typhoid, which he caught from drinking asylum water and that he was improperly treated by the medical officer, a locum, whom she alleged had treated him for influenza, instead of typhoid. The Visiting Committee had been advised by their legal counsel that they had a good defence and they agreed to proceed with the action. Before the trial was set, however, a new epidemic of typhoid broke out in the same ward as the 1906 one. All the drains and sanitary arrangements were checked and found to be in good condition. The patients were being kept in isolation and the ward disinfected. The Committee, however, decided that in view of the legal action pending the water should not be analysed.[10]

The action was tried in March 1908 by Special Jury in the High Court of King's Bench before Mr Justice Grantham. The jury found the Committee negligent in the management of the water supply, their negligence causing the water to be contaminated with sewage. The doctor was exonerated from all claims of mistreatment. The Committee was ordered to pay £650 damages and costs. Owing to the length of the trial, the necessity for expert scientific testimony and expenses of the witnesses and counsel, the hospital was forced to pay another £1850, which depleted the hospital's financial reserves, putting them in an overdraft position by having to draw on the treasurer's bond funds. The Visiting Committee immediately appealed to the County Councils for reimbursement of the £2500 'in order that the financial arrangements of the asylum may not be disorganised'.[11] The Committee applied to the Court of Appeal for either a dismissal of the verdict or a new trial, in spite of the advice from their legal counsel that they had little chance of success. Since the judgement was under appeal, the original award was held in trust. Brown's widow petitioned for interim support, and the Committee agreed to pay her three pounds per week, which would be treated as a gratuity if the appeal succeeded.[12] However, the Court of Appeal dismissed the application for a new trial. The Committee had the costs reassessed by the courts, but were not awarded any reductions, and immediately appealed the assessment which was again lost.

The three councils were asked to reimburse the asylum according to the number of beds to which each county was entitled. The counties objected, claiming that, since the farm bailiff had been paid out of the maintenance fund and as there were sufficient funds in that account, the costs should also be paid from it. Since they had no alternative, the Visiting Committee agreed to payment from the maintenance fund; with the added fees of the appeal claim, costs now totalled £3723. In order to rebuild the maintenance fund, the Committee immediately voted to increase the weekly rate of maintenance per patient charged to the County Councils from 9/4 to 10/6, thus effectively forcing them to pay.

Once the trial was over, the Committee immediately ordered a new bacteriological analysis of the asylum water supply and Stevenson reported that the water was of the 'highest purity'. Unlike the earlier test, in this case the Committee resolved that the results of the bacteriological analyses be added to their annual report to the Commissioners in Lunacy. They further resolved to have the well water tested three times in the next year and the drainage system tested twice.[13]

At the request of the medical superintendent, however, this was altered to have the next sample taken from the taps in the asylum, rather than from the wells. The tap water was found to be 'a quite satisfactory drinking water'.[14] The water supply remained a potential source of contamination and was carefully monitored. In 1911 another outbreak of typhoid occurred with twelve cases and two deaths, one attendant and one patient. The medical superintendent assured the Visiting Committee that the source of the outbreak was almost certainly not the water or milk supply. However, the bacteriological tests showed slight contamination, though the Committee registered little consternation at this result.[15]

Owing to the high number of cases of tuberculosis in the asylum, it was suggested in 1907 that the asylum cows be tested for bovine tuberculosis. The medical superintendent wrote to the department of agriculture about testing procedures. The reply warned that the test should only be administered by qualified practitioners under strict segregative conditions, with very careful handling of the tuberculin used for the test. When asked if there was any danger to human beings from cows suffering from tuberculosis 'both as regards the consumption of their milk and flesh', the Royal Veterinary College advised that milk from cows suffering from tuberculosis was a means of transmission to humans and should not be used in any form in human food.[16] The Visiting Committee decided to postpone further action and in 1909 again the motion to have the asylum herd tested was defeated. Instead it was agreed to hire a veterinarian to examine all 36 of the asylum cows and test only those which he suspected were suffering from tuberculosis – neither those that were obviously tubercular nor those that showed no signs of the disease.[17] The examination resulted in the discovery of five milking cows whose udders showed tuberculous nodules and whose milk was likely to be infectious and two others that were found positive when tested. It was recommended that all cows purchased in future be examined for signs of tuberculosis before purchase and that all those currently affected be destroyed. A programme of twice yearly

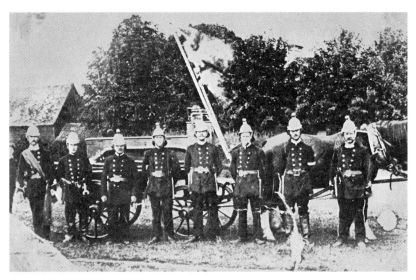

Figure 3.2 Fire brigade, c.1900

clinical inspection of the herd was undertaken, with tuberculin testing to be done only in the case of uncertainty.

Aside from infectious diseases, safety was a big concern, particularly as the use of gas lamps and open fireplaces made the threat of fire a constant source of worry. Chimney fires were not uncommon and great efforts were made to see that all chimneys were regularly cleaned. Fires did, however, break out occasionally. In 1902 there was a major fire in the east water tower. It was first noticed by the gardener, who saw smoke coming from between the slates in the roof. The fire was not extinguished for four hours after various methods had been tried and failed. The water hydrant was found to lack sufficient water pressure for the hose to reach the flames, and one of the two available engines was under repair. Efforts at putting the fire out from inside the building were found to be too dangerous and it was eventually extinguished from the higher roof of the adjoining tower. By that time, the whole roof had fallen in and the adjoining dormitories were affected. Patients had to be moved but there was no 'excitement or panic' among them. The cause was determined to be burning soot falling on the lead gutters and burning through to the rooms below. Similar fires had occurred a number of times before – in 1881, 1883 and 1894 – in different parts of the roof. De Lisle commended the efforts of the fire brigade in spite of the 'height of the situation of the fire, the difficulty in getting at it, and bringing a sufficient power of water to bear upon it' and remarked that their new helmets 'were of great service and prevented some serious wounds from falling slates and timbers'.[18]

Death of the Brewer

The most notorious incident in the hospital in the pre-war years was the drowning of the asylum brewer in a vat of beer. De Lisle reported to the Visiting Committee that Cornelius Charlie Prime, the brewer, aged 32, was found dead on 26 March 1906. An inquest was held on 29 March with the conclusion of accidental death by drowning in a vat of beer. There was no evidence to show how the accident had happened, but the Visiting Committee were much exercised by the fact that the brewer's body had not been found for forty hours, even though the brewery workers had been at their regular duties between the death and the discovery of the body. The chairman initiated an investigation and made his report.

The brewer was considered to lead a somewhat secluded life and worked independently of the steward, who was his supervisor. It seemed surprising that Prime was not missed at mealtimes and that his unused bed had gone unobserved. The mealtime absence was accounted for by the fact that the brewer took his meals with the hall porter and since the brewer often took short leave with the steward's permission, the hall porter had not considered it necessary to remark on Prime's absence. Prime's bed was made by a patient and apparently the patient had not had 'sense enough' to remark on the fact that it had not been slept in.

Prime's absence was only discovered when Thompson, the engineer, wanted the use of the brewery engine and went looking for Prime, who could not be found. The hall porter told Thompson that Prime must be away on leave. Thompson consulted the steward who said that Prime was not on leave and, on making a search of the brewery, discovered the body. The other unanswered question was how the brewery workers were let into the brewery buildings if Prime, who held the keys, was not there to open the doors for them. It was discovered that Prime had arranged with the storekeeper to let the workers in at 8 am so that he would not have to get up so early. The storekeeper advised the chairman that he was not aware there were regulations to the contrary.

At the inquest, the steward reported that, on hearing Prime could not be found, he went to his bedroom and found that Prime's bed had not been slept in. He next checked to see if Prime's keys were in his office at the brewery, which would alert him as to whether Prime was on the premises or not. As the keys were missing, he assumed Prime must be around. He searched the brewery and found nothing until he reached the vat room. He looked in all three vats, and in the third saw something that resembled a sack, but when he tried to lift it, found it was a man's leg. The body could not be moved and some attendants were called to help. The only way to remove the body was to drain the vat from below. There were 400 gallons of beer in the five-and-a-half-foot diameter vat. The beer was four and a half feet deep, including four inches of yeast in which the brewer's cap was floating. When the vat was drained, Prime's body was found with his head under one of the coils and a foot entangled in another.

Prime had worked as the brewer for eight years and was the keeper of the keys to the brewery. It was his job to take the temperature of the vats, which he did on Monday afternoons. One of the patients working in the brewery stated that Prime had taken him into the brewery at three o'clock and had left him downstairs washing barrels. There were three patients working in the brewery, none of whom were considered to have homicidal tendencies. Prime's watch was stopped at 3.42, and the asylum medical officer who examined Prime's body found no signs of a struggle. He concluded that Prime had died from drowning after having been overcome by fumes which caused him to fall into the vat.[19]

Mental Defectives and Criminal Lunatics

The first patients classified as criminally insane were admitted to TCA in 1911. There had been much debate by the Visiting Committee, who feared that having what were considered to be dangerous patients might be disruptive to other patients and create difficulties for the staff. However, they received payment for them from the Prison Commissioners above the rate for regular pauper lunatic patients and saw the potential for additional income. By August 1911, the asylum had taken in fourteen criminal lunatic patients, eight men and six women 'of a quiet class'. Further transfers were made in the next year until a total of 28 prisoners were in the asylum. Occasionally, when a prison sentence had been served and the prisoner was considered unfit for discharge, he or she would be transferred to the regular pauper class, providing they were originally from one of the three counties. In 1913 all but one of the 28 prisoners were transferred to Broadmoor and no more were received until after the war.

In May 1919 the Visiting Committee received a letter from the Home Office stating that with the great reduction in criminal lunatics they could no longer justify keeping two asylums, Rampton and Broadmoor, for strictly criminal cases. Rampton was to be converted to an institution for mental defectives who were considered dangerous or violent, and some of the criminal lunatics then housed in Rampton were to be transferred to county and borough asylums, with the remainder going to Broadmoor. To make room for them, it would be necessary to transfer some patients whose condition meant that they could reasonably be housed in local asylums. These would be patients who had been charged with serious crimes, but were not considered dangerous.

The Visiting Committee advised the Home Office that they could take 90 male and 40 female prisoners. By December 1919 the Prison Commissioners were ready to start sending patients and in January 66 male and nineteen female criminal lunatics were admitted. The following month the Committee reported that they had taken another 21 female criminals and 44 males from Broadmoor, making a total of 150 criminal lunatics who were being kept under special observation (twenty more than the Visiting Committee had originally suggested) and who seemed 'appeased, quiet and orderly'.[20] By September 1921 there were still 138 criminal patients, but by 1922 the majority of these had been transferred back to Broadmoor.[21]

Under the 1913 Act, institutions for the mentally defective were to be small and educationally oriented, rather than medical establishments. Inmates were to be protected from exploitation and, given the popularity of the eugenics movement, segregated by sex to avoid the possibility of defective offspring. Under the same act, the Lunacy Commission was replaced by the Board of Control who were responsible for both mental illness and mental deficiency.[22]

The Visiting Committee proposed to use the Wilbury Farm property as a home for mental defectives and decided to approach the Board of Control for approval.[23] It was also necessary to get the three counties to approve and to send their mental defectives to TCA before the Committee considered converting the buildings.[24] This was finally agreed in 1922 and approval was given to start the work.

After the war there was renewed movement towards categorising and separating patients within the mentally ill classification. In 1921, the Board of Control declared that they were pleased with TCA's efforts in classifying patients according to their mental state. The only thing they noted was the absence of separate accommodation for acute cases who were quiet and possibly recoverable. These patients were then put in with new admissions of all types and some chronic cases. It was arranged with staff that Ward 7 on both the male and female sides of the hospital be adapted for the purpose, as they were bright and well-furnished and 'this class of patient seems to merit the best accommodation'.[25]

Death Rates, Post Mortems and the Pathology Laboratory

The Lunacy Commissioners' report for 1894 complained of the high death rate in the asylum compared to other asylums. The Visiting Committee responded that the death rate was only marginally higher, being 11.00 per 1000 average for the previous five years compared with the national asylum average of 10.11 per 1000. The explanation for the higher rate was that TCA took in an inordinately large number of elderly patients. The Commissioners had made special mention of the large number dying from tuberculosis and pneumonia, seventeen and nine respectively in 1894. The Committee noted that three of the pneumonia patients were over 70. Of the consumptive patients, two had the disease on admission and the others 'betrayed a tendency towards it'. The report also recommended that the spare coffins be removed from the post-mortem room to the cemetery tool house, and that rods and curtains be provided to give more privacy when friends of the deceased came to view the bodies.[26] The lack of a pathology laboratory was also noted, with the added comment that, if one were to be provided, the doctors might 'take more interest in this area of scientific research'. The pathology laboratory was finally constructed in 1914, in a room formerly used as a clock room next to the medical superintendent's office.[27]

The Commissioners regularly cited inefficiencies in record-keeping, particularly the pathological records and case books, and the conducting of post-mortem examinations. The Visiting Committee, however, felt that the records were being kept as they should but that perhaps the notes on chronic cases were too short. To the recommendation that post mortems be done in all cases of death in the hospital, the Committee responded that in many cases friends and family objected to the procedure and in others, according to the medical superintendent, there was thought to be nothing to be gained by it. The Visiting Committee recommended that if the Commissioners desired that clinical records be kept as in regular hospitals for case notes and pathological records, then another assistant medical officer would have to be hired to handle the extra workload.[28] Eventually, in the new version of the rules and regulations for the asylum produced in 1924, a stipulation was included that a post-mortem examination be done on every patient who died in the asylum.[29]

The original burial ground for the asylum had been consecrated in 1864 by the Bishop of Ely. By 1897, the cemetery was estimated to have about 2000 graves of patients, each marked with a small wooden or iron cross and numbered for reference.[30] Additional burial-ground space was soon needed and the Visiting Committee obtained the necessary approvals from the counties, the Lunacy Commissioners and the diocese offices and had the new ground consecrated, though the ceremony was much less elaborate than the original consecration.

Improved Working Conditions for Staff

During the period 1900–1925, working life improved significantly for asylum staff. The installation of an internal telephone system in 1891 had reduced the long treks between wards and buildings. In 1906, the Visiting Committee agreed to have an external telephone system installed by the General Post Office at an initial cost of £60 plus additional fees for calls. The telephone poles were to go through the asylum property from the Stotfold road to Arlesey village. The Stotfold exchange opened in August 1907 and the asylum was awaiting the opening of the Arlesey exchange. The Post Office agreed to supply the asylum with the necessary 'instruments' for a fee of £5, which would entitle the asylum to 500 calls per year. Additional calls would be charged at 1d per call for any call made in the Hitchin exchange area. The Committee emphasised the need for 'strict secrecy' on the part of the exchange operators, due to the nature of the institution. The Committee also urged the County of Bedford to connect the various police stations in Bedfordshire to the exchange, as had already been done in Hertford and Huntingdon, to aid in the capture of escaped patients.[31] In January 1908 the asylum telephone system was in full running order and a number of police stations in Bedfordshire had been connected.

In 1909 the Asylum Officers' Superannuation Act was passed, enabling staff to have a regular contributory pension plan. Prior to the Act, all staff had to apply on retiring to the Visiting Committee to be granted a pension. Approval for the pension and its amount was entirely at the discretion of the Committee, who had to apply to the county councils for approval under the 1890 Lunacy Act. Amounts granted for female attendants were only a fraction of that of male attendants. With the passing of the Superannuation Act, male and female attendants got equal treatment for pensions, but since women's earnings were significantly lower than men's, their pensions were correspondingly small. The Committee were obliged to draw up a scheme for implementation of the Act before it came into force in April 1910. Prior to the Act, a whole group of tradespeople were not entitled to a pension, as they were not considered permanent employees of the asylum. This group included a tailor's assistant who had been working at the asylum for 29 years, a labourer who had been employed for eighteen years, and a bricklayer with fifteen years' service. For the purposes of assigning contributions and payments, the Committee divided the asylum staff into two classes, the first class for those who were directly responsible for patients, and the second class for those who were not. Since patients were engaged in work in all parts of the asylum, the number of those who had no responsibilities for patients was small, limited mainly to assistant tradesmen and labourers.[32]

In early 1910 the Committee received an application from the asylum attendants for a money allowance in lieu of beer. This was not the first time this request had been brought before the Committee. In the original petition in 1902, the attendants claimed that the money would be more beneficial and more helpful to them than the beer. The idea had been consistently rejected out of hand as being too expensive, and also because it would necessitate the closure of the brewery. Male attendants were allowed two and a half pints of beer daily and female attendants one pint. The argument against closing the brewery was that the cost to the asylum of supplying beer was just over £500 per year, including a daily glass of beer for patients. In 1910, if the attendants were to be paid the equivalent of what it would cost to buy the beer, it would amount to £600 per annum and the patients would be deprived of their beer through the closing of the brewery. This, the medical superintendent felt, might bring on a strike by the working patients, particularly those engaged in hard manual labour. If the patients were deprived of their beer, other changes might then have to be made, possibly to the daily diet, or for extra tobacco which would have to be purchased. The Committee narrowly voted to reject the attendants' application.[33]

A month later, de Lisle tendered his resignation on the grounds of ill health, after serving 29 years in the asylum, ten of those as medical superintendent. The advertisement for a new superintendent was placed in *The Lancet* and the *British Medical Journal*.[34] Laurence Otway Fuller was appointed in August 1910 and within a short time introduced a number of changes.

Fuller supported the closing of the brewery when the question of attendants being given money in lieu of a beer allowance came up

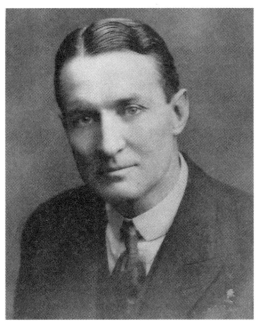

Figure 3.3 Laurence Otway Fuller, Medical Superintendent, c. 1920

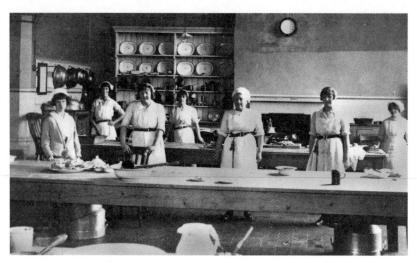

Figure 3.4 Kitchen staff, c. 1920

again in 1911. At the same time, attendants all over the country were petitioning for a shorter working week to be legislated, which would limit the working hours of asylum attendants to 140 per fortnight. The Visiting Committee, hoping to avert the reduced work week, which would cause considerable expense in hiring additional staff, finally acceded to the request to give up the beer allowance. Unlike de Lisle, Fuller made no remonstrance about the patients' loss of their beer allotment. In fact, consideration of the patients did not enter the discussion in 1911. In lieu of their daily beer allowance, it was agreed to pay £3 to each male attendant and £2 to each female attendant and farm servant per year. There was also a provision made for the attendants to purchase mineral water at the rate of two bottles per day, for the sum of 10/- annually. The asylum staff did not risk drinking the tap water, though presumably the patients had no choice. At the same time as they approved the money allowance, the Visiting Committee agreed to close the brewery and all stocks of hops and malt were sold off.[35] Plans were made for the brewery to be converted to a bakery and bacon factory.

Fuller was intolerant of the abuse of patients by staff and several attendants were dismissed for such incidents during his tenure as superintendent. The first of these was only a month after his appointment. Fuller reported that a patient had complained of being assaulted by an attendant. On interviewing the patient and some witnesses, it was determined that the attendant was at fault. He was dismissed and legal action was taken against him at the Biggleswade Petty Sessions. Three patients, Fuller, and one of the assistant medical officers gave evidence. The attendant was convicted and fined £2.[36] A few months later an attendant was dismissed, with a month's notice, for using bad language to a patient, which Fuller had overheard. In the same month, Fuller investigated rumours of immoral behaviour between a married male and single female attendant who, when interrogated, 'practically admitted the truth of the rumour'. They were dismissed on the spot and ordered to leave the asylum at once.[37] On one occasion when a patient had committed suicide, Fuller considered the charge attendant partially to blame and demoted him to ordinary attendant. Any hint of drink among attendants while on duty was dealt with severely, and several were dismissed during Fuller's tenure for showing signs of intoxication. Similarly, on more than one occasion when a patient escaped, attendants were held responsible and either demoted or dismissed, depending on the seriousness of their presumed negligence.

One important change initiated by Fuller led to more accuracy in keeping patient records. Fuller explained to the Committee that it was often difficult, when patients were first admitted, to diagnose the form of mental illness from which they were suffering. It took time to assess the patient's condition, which sometimes only became apparent after a period of observation. Under the regulations, the admissions registers had to be submitted to the Committee every month, with the diagnoses filled in and copies sent to the Commissioners in Lunacy. The result was often that the diagnosis changed after observation and

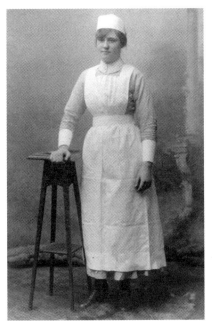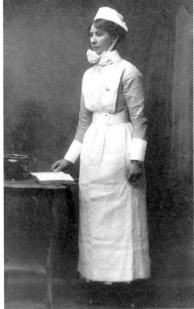

Figure 3.5 Uniformed nursing staff

thus the registers and the Commissioners' records became incorrect. On consideration, the Committee agreed with Fuller that the diagnosis should not in future have to be put in the register until it was properly ascertained.[38]

During the First World War, the movement to improve working conditions for staff, including the institution of an asylum workers' union, continued, but the shortages of staff and resources prevented any real gains. Immediately after the War, however, the movement gained momentum, and in December 1918 the Asylum Workers' Union was recognised by the Visiting Committee.[39] The following month the Committee received a letter from the National Asylum Workers' Union, asking for increases in salary, a reduction in working hours and other concessions.[40] An industrial tribunal was subsequently set up by the London County Council to consider the union's requests, and the Visiting Committee, following London's lead, began an internal review process which, after some delaying tactics by the Committee, resulted in a shorter working week and wage increases for all staff.[41]

The First World War

Between the outbreak of war in August 1914 and March 1915, 24 TCA staff had enlisted and three had been killed in action. In June 1915, the Board of Control asked the hospital to release a medical officer to work in a new hospital being set up for treating wounded soldiers, but the Committee refused, as the asylum was already very short staffed. Also during 1915, asylums were canvassed to see how many beds could be made available for the treatment of wounded soldiers. TCA offered up to 100 beds, but before the offer was acted upon a new system was devised, whereby the country was divided into eight regions, and one asylum in each region was to be set aside entirely for military patients. In the TCA region, Norfolk Asylum was vacated for the purpose and over the next three years TCA took over 350 Norfolk patients.

Prices rose steadily during the war, with shortages brought on by resources being redirected to the war effort. Within months of the war starting, contractors supplying the hospital put their prices up dramatically, even on existing contracts, and the Visiting Committee sought legal advice, with the result that they took on new contracts for a short time period, thinking that the war might be over quickly. With the introduction of rationing in 1917, the hospital made even greater efforts towards self-sufficiency and began producing their own cheese. An example of the increase in prices driven by war shortages is the rise in maintenance costs of patients. Private patients who had been paying between 15/- and 20/- per week upkeep at the beginning of the war were being charged 35/- to 42/- by 1923.

At the outbreak of the war, the Visiting Committee agreed to allow staff to enlist, providing the safety of the asylum was not jeopardised and temporary staff could be hired to fill in. The Committee also agreed to supplement army pay to equal their salary as attendants. The first TCA employee to be killed in action was Arthur Titmus in November of 1914, followed by W. Brandram in December, William Ellis in March 1915, and Frank Fowler the following September. The Committee prepared a roll of honour for employees serving in the war and hung it in 'a conspicuous place' in the main building. By 1916 so many staff had enlisted that the asylum was using tradespeople as temporary attendants. The Visiting Committee applied to the Board of Control to get exemption for attendants, which was granted on a temporary basis. The Committee also agreed to take on conscientious objectors as attendants if they were deemed suitable as employees.

The War Office regularly appealed for doctors from the asylum to enlist, but the Committee consistently refused, saying they were already very short staffed. By 1917 they were ordered by the Board of Control to send one medical officer and Dr Hunter, who had earlier been considered too old for active service, was sent. Dr Gavin, one of the junior medical officers who had signed up at the beginning of the war, was awarded the Military Cross in June 1917, but in November was killed in France when he was thrown from his horse and suffered a fractured skull. After the invasion of Belgium by Germany in October 1914 around a quarter of a million refugees came over to the UK for the duration of the war. The government specified that town boards up and down the country should make provision to accommodate the influx and meet their many needs. Large institutions such as TCA were expected to play their part too in offering free care where necessary and the hospital began to take in Belgian refugees. A concert was also staged in the dining hall to raise money for the refugee fund. The refugees were not considered paupers but were classed as private patients for whom the Board of Control was to be billed directly.

Shell-shock

In the first months of the war there was little public awareness of a condition that was to become endemic among soldiers serving at the front. A hint of what was to come was evident in the application of one of the asylum's medical officers for leave to take a position as house physician in the National Hospital for Nervous Diseases in London, where he hoped to become acquainted with modern methods of treatment.[42] In 1916 the Visiting Committee received a request from the Board of Control to take discharged soldiers and sailors who suffered from mental disorders brought on by service in the war. The War Office was anxious that they not be classified as paupers and suffer the stigma that attached to that label. Their pensions would more than cover the maintenance costs and it was requested that a new category of 'service patients' be created for them and that they be classified as private patients in the registers. If they were to be kept with other patients they were to be allowed to wear a distinctive uniform or badge.[43] Service patients dying in the asylum were not to be buried in the asylum cemetery, and a contract for £5 was to be entered into with a local undertaker for burial in the local parish cemetery.[44]

Shell-shock or war neurosis was a highly controversial and contested diagnosis. The War Office was not eager to recognise it for several reasons. Besides depleting the troops and undermining morale, there was the economic factor of providing lifelong pensions for so many young men. From a medical and military perspective, initially it was seen as malingering and cowardice and there was a call for court martialling. In extreme cases, shell-shocked soldiers were shot as deserters, but at home both Parliament and the public were becoming increasingly sympathetic and private charities were set up to support sufferers. By 1917 the numbers were so great, wholesale court martial would have been impossible. Added to the strength of public sympathy, there was eventually a grudging acceptance that it might be a medical condition requiring treatment.

Originally special hospitals had been created or appropriated for treatment of shell-shocked patients, but as the war progressed the numbers grew until it was estimated that there were up to 80,000 cases. Between 1919 and 1939, 114,000 ex-servicemen suffering from war-related neurasthenia made applications to the Ministry of Pensions.[45] The few designated hospitals could never cope with these numbers. There was a chronic shortage of beds and it was inevitable that the county asylums would end up sharing the care costs for ex-servicemen in their communities.

In 1917 TCA began to admit soldiers suffering from shell-shock. Most of them were transferred from military hospitals at Warrington, Napsbury and Netley. On admission, they were transferred to the private-patient class as 'service patients'. Between August 1917 and January 1920, 77 were admitted to TCA. None were from the officer class. Most were listed as gunners, sappers and privates. Some had been discharged and were admitted from their home town rather than the war hospitals.[46]

Patients suffering from shell-shock were diagnosed according to the Schedule of Forms of Insanity (see appendix, p. 115) as suffering from 'confusional insanity'. A typical case is that of D.H., a 36-year-old ex-soldier who was transferred from the Crookston War Hospital in Glasgow to TCA in 1918. Ex-servicemen were normally transferred from war hospitals to a hospital in their local county. D.H. had been in France and had been sick for nine months. He was described on admission as becoming progressively dull, apathetic and easily confused. His memory for recent events was faulty, and his memory of events in France was a complete blank. He described himself as feeling shaky and said his head felt as though it was swimming around. Although he had no hallucinations or delusions, he was slow and hesitating in answering questions and seemed confused. The medical superintendent noted that 'he is said to have had shell-shock'. Monthly case notes indicate a progressive recovery. He began to talk more coherently, his memory improved, he began to work well, and he became more cheerful and interested. However, his memory of events in France remained blank. Within eight months he was discharged on trial in the care of his wife and did not re-enter the hospital.[47]

A similar case was A.C., aged 22, who was admitted in September 1918. He had been at Lord Derby's War Hospital at Warrington and was discharged in December 1917. He had joined the army soon after the war started and was wounded at Gallipoli. At Cairo he got sunstroke and was invalided home. He subsequently recovered, went to France 'and suffered from "shell-shock" in which he lost his speech, which came back to him suddenly in a Picture Palace'. He displayed much the same symptoms as D.H., especially with regard to having little recall of events in France. He was also incoherent and complained of waking up in a state of fear. His illness was of a much shorter duration, recorded as being of three days' duration on his admission to TCA. He was discharged, recovered, within three months.[48]

Less optimistic cases were those of soldiers who were admitted suffering from shell-shock complicated by a tendency towards, or explicitly suffering from, another form of mental illness. These cases often never recovered and died in hospital. One such case was H.S., a private, who was admitted at age 34 in 1918. The description of his mental state on admission was typical of severely shell-shocked cases. The admission notes state:

> His attention can be gained but it is difficult to retain it for any lengthy conversation. He answers simple questions fairly well but hesitatingly and very soon lapses into a state of […] confusion. He has no idea at all of his surroundings, time or date and is not fully aware of his own identity and also mistakes that of people around him. His comprehension, associativity of ideas, and reasoning powers

are at a very low ebb and his memory for recent as well as remote events is markedly impaired. He talks incoherently, wandering from one subject to another most disjointedly. He has distinct auditory and visual hallucinations with various imaginary people, [he] also sees them but is unable to describe what they are like. He also appears to have a few delusions of an exalted type, such as being the subject of especial persecution.[49]

Within two years his condition had deteriorated and mental deficiency was added to his form of insanity along with confusional insanity. He had become violent and destructive and by the 1930s was completely mute and 'quite demented'. By 1947 he was described as 'dirty, untidy, unemployable and unchanged'. He died in 1948 of dysentery and pneumonia after thirty years in TCA.

C.M., a sapper with the Royal Engineers, was admitted in 1915 aged 29. Although he was not explicitly a shell-shock sufferer, his case is interesting as it illustrates the cultural relativity of delusional states. While patients suffering from delusions of grandeur often consider themselves either religious or royal personages, C.M.'s delusions were mainly war-related. After serving at Flanders and a number of other battles, he had fallen into a trench and severely injured his back. He was invalided to hospital and eventually discharged home, where he began to suffer from extreme delusional states. On admission, he was considered very violent and unstable. He demanded that everyone call him the 'All Div', short for the 'All Divine', and insisted he could close heaven to anyone who crossed him. He considered himself the 'hero of heroes', claiming he had saved thousands of men's lives, had seven Victoria Crosses, had shot down an aeroplane and obtained all the plans of the German campaign. A year after admission he was considered very unstable, suffering from delusional insanity and maintaining his delusions of being a war hero. Within five years of his admission he caught typhoid and died in the hospital in 1920.[50]

These cases are typical of the thousands of ex-soldiers who were discharged into county mental hospitals. The public outcry and sympathy for them brought the treatment of mental illness into the public sphere and divested it of some of its secrecy and stigma. The importance of shell-shock treatment to the subsequent development of therapies for the mentally ill cannot be underestimated. Before the war there was little effort to develop active therapeutic regimes. Asylums still operated predominantly on the basis of moral treatment. Efforts at treating the thousands of shell-shocked soldiers opened up possibilities for treatment that were to radically alter the world view of mental illness and the potential for curative therapies.

J.R.

Non-military patients at TCA were well aware of the war and those who were able made their own contributions in small ways. One female patient, J.R., wrote patriotic poetry which was privately printed by her sister. J.R., a domestic servant, had been admitted to the asylum at age 36 in 1908 suffering from chronic melancholia. She was described on admission as being 'very strange in manner, restless, throwing herself about on the bed or floor, refusing to speak or answer questions, but calling out occasionally at the top of her voice "What Sir". She refuses her food and can only be got to take a little milk by persuasion. She is dirty in her habits.'[51]

J.R.'s case notes were not regularly kept until 1912, when the system for individual case notes was instituted. For most of 1912 she had settled down and was working in the laundry. She was considered improved and working well, though sometimes depressed and given to bouts of crying. It was noted that she blamed her upbringing for her condition, saying she had been spoilt and pampered. By March of 1913, however, she had relapsed and become dazed and excited, rushing about 'with her dress disordered and her hair down and repeating everything which was said to her and repeatedly crossing herself before the pictures in the ward; said she could hear her sister calling to her. When given a book to read spelt out every word.' After this episode she continued to improve and within six months was reported to be working well in the medical superintendent's house. By the end of the year her sister appeared before the Visiting Committee stating that J.R. wished to be discharged and that she was prepared to take her. The medical superintendent cautioned that she would have to be kept under constant and close observation for two months. Her sister could not guarantee this and her petition was refused. In November 1916 J.R. was described as being 'very exalted and constantly asking to go home; is clean and tidy; has developed a poetic inspiration and has lately had one of her effusions printed by her sister'. Her sister subsequently printed several of J.R.'s war poems, which were strongly patriotic and remarkably lucid given her mental state (see below).

By 1918 J.R. was considered well enough to go home on a two-month trial and was discharged into the care of her sister. Within a month she was back, in a very agitated state, throwing herself about the room, exposing herself and singing and talking excitedly. This cycle of mania and melancholia repeated itself throughout the war years: at times J.R. was classed as an excellent worker, keeping quiet for months at a time with only the occasional off day, then she would relapse into a manic state. Ultimately J.R.'s dread of never being released from the hospital was realised. She died of cardiac failure in the asylum in 1933 at the age of 62.

The Post-war Era

Dr Hunter wrote to the Visiting Committee in May 1919, requesting that he be demobilised and returned to duties at the hospital. The Committee quickly sent a letter to the Board of Control requesting Hunter's 'speedy release'.[52] The Ministry of Labour sent requests to all asylums asking that ex-servicemen be employed whenever possible. The Visiting Committee agreed to hire them when the occasion arose and when suitable.[53] The Minister of Pensions began a scheme for separating the service patients from ordinary mental patients and sent the Inspector of Service Patients to TCA to see about possible sites. Wilbury Farm was proposed though the plan was not pursued. By 1922 there were still 29 service patients who were warded together with the male private patients. The Visiting Committee remarked that the ex-servicemen seemed contented and were 'receiving privileges due to their class'.[54]

Within a year of the war ending, the question of a private patients' scheme was again considered. In 1919 it was agreed that alterations be made to the east and west ends of the asylum main building for private accommodation. The dormitories would include partitioned cubicles for privacy, though this was later found to take up too much space and the partitions were changed to screens.[55] The plans were finally approved by the Board of Control in October 1919, and the new accommodation was called East View and West View. The Committee drew up an advertisement to be placed in the local papers in the three counties, a daily paper and the medical papers to read as follows:

> Special accommodation for Private Patients of both sexes is provided at 'East View' and 'West View'. Ample provision is made for treatment, occupation and entertainment of the Patients. The situation is high and rural and the air bracing. Terms 35/- per week, including all necessaries, except clothing and stimulants. Further particulars and Form of Admission may be obtained on application to the Medical Superintendent.[56]

The weekly rate was to be made up of the current rate for pauper patients plus 5/- weekly rent to the counties for the accommodation per patient and 7/10 as an extra charge for better conditions. If desired, a private room could be provided for 7/- extra per week.[57] By July 1920 the private accommodation was ready to receive patients and the advertisements were placed in the papers. Within a year, there were 68 private patients in the hospital, though not all would have been accommodated in East and West View. About 30 of these were ex-servicemen who were grouped with the other male private patients.

The chaplain, Rev. A. Atkinson, resigned in late 1918, just as the war ended. He had been hospital chaplain since 1902 and was leaving to take up a living in Loxley, Lincolnshire.[58] The new chaplain, the Rev. R. La Porte-Payne, was appointed in October 1918. Under his direction, a memorial window in the east end of the chapel was to be installed in honour of hospital employees who had been killed in the war. Permission was given by the Visiting Committee for a public concert to be held in the hospital to raise funds for the window.[59] Patients became involved in the fundraising as well. J.R. wrote a poem in support:

For our War Memorial

Well, friends, the war is over,
Peace is signed they say,
But many of our brave lads
In foreign graves now lay,
And it would be a shame, friends,
If we, in selfishness,
Should let it be forgotten
How they have died for us;
And as we cannot place a stone
Above each noble man,
Let's gladly join together,
And do the best we can.
Let us in our Church here,
A lovely window raise,
When children and when visitors,
Upon that picture gaze,
How gladly shall we say to them,
The window that you see
Was raised here by the T.C.A.,
In loving memory.

J.R.
July 1919

A year later the chaplain had the opportunity to purchase a window of pre-war workmanship and material for £100 of which £65 had already been raised. The Visiting Committee agreed to donate £25 towards the cost and requested that they approve the wording for the memorial. It was unveiled by the Chairman of the Visiting Committee on 31 May 1920.

The main effect of the war on asylum life was the development of new therapies and the growing realisation that mental illness could be treated. Although the new treatment regimes were not actively adopted at TCA until the 1930s, the recognition that successful treatment was a possibility began to take hold in the early post-war years. Since 1900, asylum attendants had been offered a rudimentary training programme by the Medico-Psychological Association. This organisation had been formed in 1865, out of the Association of Medical Officers of Asylums for the Insane.[60] At TCA attendants were encouraged to pursue certification, and on completion of the programme were awarded pay increases. The Association was not very progressive and its emphasis in training attendants was largely on the mental-health legislation rather than active therapies. Within the Association there was substantial resistance to the new therapies for shell-shock, with their psychoanalytic orientation.[61] At TCA, although non-mental ailments were routinely treated where treatments existed, the first mention in the asylum records (in the Annual Report of the Visiting Committee for 1919) of a systematic treatment for mental illness was the possibility of using psychoanalysis. The Visiting Committee agreed in 1921 to provide financial help and other facilities to enable medical officers to take up special courses of instruction. One of the junior medical officers took the examinations and was granted study leave by the Committee. There is, however, little reference in the hospital records to any active treatments up to the mid-1920s. Asylum finances were run on a strict budget and any extra expenditure was scrutinised closely for its overall benefit. No real changes were undertaken either in the physical fabric of the hospital or in treatment regimes unless there was a very strong case for them. This meant that the hospital was slow to adopt new therapies and would only consider them if there was substantial evidence that they had worked in other asylums, or there was legislation that required compliance.

The dramatic changes in the social fabric of British society after the war were slow to penetrate the closed world of the asylum, but they began to in the 1920s with a change in terminology. In 1921 the Visiting Committee received a letter from the Cambridgeshire County Asylum recommending that the terms 'pauper lunatic' and 'pauper lunatic asylum' be discontinued and that the Ministry of Health be asked to amend the Lunacy Act by substituting 'patients' and 'hospital'. The Fulbourn committee urged TCA to pass their own resolution to that effect. In 1927, authority was received from the Ministry to adopt the new terminology and the asylum officially changed its name to Three Counties Hospital (TCH). The name change heralded an era of modernisation, much of which was directly or indirectly linked to changes effected by the war.

Notes

1   LF4/1/1b, Committee of Visitors, Minutes of Visit, 26 May 1896.
2   LF3/2, Epitomes, 26 July 1909.
3   LF3/3, 27 Feb 1911.
4   *Ibid.*, 18 Dec 1911.
5   LF4/1/1b, Nov 1894.
6   LF3/2, 26 May 1902.
7   Ibid., 21 Jan 1907.
8   LF3/2, Minutes of Special Meeting of the Visiting Committee, 2 Oct 1906.
9   LF3/2, 29 Oct 1906.
10   *Ibid.*, 20 Jan 1908.
11   LT6/9, Special Report from the Visiting Committee to the County Councils of Bedford, Hertford and Huntingdon, 27 Apr 1908.
12   LF3/2, Minutes of a Special Meeting of the Visiting Committee, 21 Apr 1908.
13   *Ibid.*, 25 May 1908.
14   LF3/2, 26 Apr 1909.
15   LF3/3, 20 Nov 1911.
16   LF3/2, 23 Dec 1907.
17   *Ibid.*, 22 Feb 1909.
18   *Ibid.*, 24 Mar 1902.
19   LF3/3, 23 Apr 1906.
20   LF1/20, 23 Feb 1920.
21   LF1/21, 26 Sept 1921, 27 Mar 1922.
22   K. Jones, *Asylums and After: A Revised History of the Mental Health Services from the Early 18th Century to the 1990s.* Athlone Press 1993, 123.
23   LF1/20, 24 Jan 1919.
24   LF1/21, 23 May 1921.
25   *Ibid.*, 25 Apr 1921.
26   LF4/1/1b, 20 June 1894.
27   LF3/3, 23 Feb 1914.
28   LF4/1/1b, 9 July 1894.
29   LT6/8, General Rules and Regulations for the Asylum, 1924.
30   LF4/1/1b, 11 Aug 1897.
31   LF3/2, 21 Oct 1907.
32   LT6/10, Asylum Officers' Superannuation Act 1909.
33   LF3/3, 25 Apr 1910.
34   *Ibid.*, 25 Jul 1910.
35   *Ibid.*, 28 Aug 1911.
36   *Ibid.*, 26 Sept and 24 Oct 1910.
37   LF3/3, 27 Feb 1911.
38   LF3/3, 27 Mar 1911.
39   LF1/20, 23 Dec 1918.
40   *Ibid.*, 24 Jan 1919.

41   *Ibid.*, 24 Feb 1919.

42   LF3/4, 21 Dec 1914.

43   Ibid., 28 Aug 1916.

44   *Ibid.*, 23 Sept 1918.

45   M. Stone, 'Shellshock and the psychologists' in W. Bynum, R. Porter and M. Shepherd, *The Anatomy of Madness: Essays in the History of Psychiatry*, Vol. II., Tavistock Publications, 1985, 242–71.

46   LF47/3, Civil Register of Private Patients, 1917–20.

47   LF32, Patient case notes.

48   *Ibid.*

49   *Ibid.*

50   *Ibid.*

51   LF33, Patient case notes.

52   LF1/20, 26 May 1919.

53   LF1/20, 22 Sept 1919.

54   LF1/21, 24 Jul 1922. In May 1959 the hospital still had eighteen patients from the 1914–18 war and ten from the 1939–45 war.

55   LF1/20, Committee of Visitors, Minutes of Monthly Meetings, 24 Apr 1919.

56   LF1/20, 24 Nov 1919.

57   *Ibid.*

58   *Ibid.*, 23 Sept 1918.

59   LF1/20, 28 Apr 1919.

60   Jones 1993, 93.

61   Stone 1985, 246–7.

CHAPTER FOUR

Modernisation, New Therapies and the NHS

The years 1930–60 saw fundamental changes in the way that Three Counties Hospital operated and essentially marked its progression from a Victorian asylum to something recognisable as a modern psychiatric facility. The main building itself remained largely unchanged throughout these years. There was little in the way of additions or demolition from the 1880s onwards and the building remained one of the best preserved Victorian asylums until its closure. New wards and facilities were built, particularly during the 1930s, but these were physically separate from the original hospital and did not much affect the look of George Fowler Jones' building.

Though the old asylum changed little, this era saw a fundamental transition from passive to active treatment regimes. The massive social upheavals generated by the First World War created a climate of experimentation and an openness to new ideas which led to changes in the structure of the mental-health system, such as the introduction of voluntary admissions in the 1930s and the creation of the NHS in the 1940s.

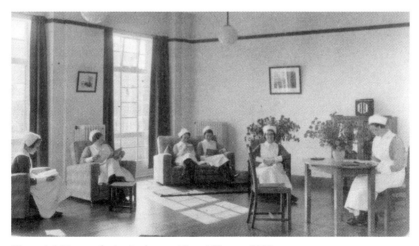

Figure 4.1 Nurses relaxing in the new Nurses' Home, c.1938

Nurses and the Nurses' Home 1925–38

From the founding of the hospital in 1860, it had been usual for male and female nursing staff to live locally and travel into work for their eleven-hour shifts. While this was acceptable to people who had homes nearby, it posed considerable difficulties when the management committee wanted to attract staff from further afield. The senior staff from the medical superintendent to the pathologist, farm bailiff, the matron, the chaplain, the secretary to the hospital and the head male nurse were all given houses or flats as part of their salary. These are generally referred to in the accounts as 'emoluments', which also meant fuel, light and laundry in most cases – although the medical superintendent also received an allowance for furniture, food and spirits.

Unmarried nursing staff had always been allowed to live in the hospital building itself, but the prospect of finding oneself in single rooms near to the patients' dormitories was never very popular as it meant that much off-duty time was spent with patients. As it became more difficult to attract staff, new solutions were sought to the problem of accommodation for unmarried female staff. The Board of Control had been urging the Visiting Committee for some years to consider building a nurses' home, a proposal the Committee considered to be unnecessarily radical and expensive. In 1924 Dr Fuller, the medical superintendent, suggested they adapt the empty isolation hospital as a staff residence. Built in 1878, it was to be converted to a residence for private patients after the war.[1] Patients with dangerous contagious diseases such as typhoid and diphtheria were sent either to Wilbury Farm or to the new isolation block built in 1923 behind the female wards.[2] The original 'butterfly-plan' isolation hospital designed by George Fowler Jones was duly divided into 22 cubicles for single female staff and opened as 'The Homestead' in late 1925. It was certainly better than living on the wards, but was judged by the Commissioners of the Board of Control as 'only partially meeting the needs which are evident in this hospital'.[3]

Working life for staff was hard by today's standards and a strict behavioural code was enforced. The medical superintendent retained draconian powers over the lives of the people who worked under him. Numerous reports from the 1860s onwards record, for example, staff being dismissed or disciplined for marrying without his permission. In the annual register of asylum staff, officers and servants for 1925 there are listed 50 male day nurses and 65 female day nurses, including charge nurses of both sexes. There were also seven male and nine female staff detailed for night duty.[4] The average wage for male nurses at that time was between 58/- and 68/- per week, with 1/6 extra for those in the asylum band, and 5/- for those who held a certificate of the Medico-

Psychological Association. The wages for female nurses were lower at 36/10 to 50/- per week, with 4/- extra for holding a certificate of qualification.

A new grade of 'probationer' nurse was created in November 1926, after the Mental Hospitals Association suggested that this might attract staff who were more career-minded and sought professional qualifications.[5] A probationer nurse was given a three-year course of training which included both academic and practical experience and led to an examination. Throughout the 1920s there had been severe difficulties in finding and keeping enough male and female nursing staff, and advertisements were often placed in newspapers in other parts of the country, most notably in the *Yorkshire Post*. This led to an influx of new staff from the North and the Midlands, which increased with the unemployment generated by the General Strike of 1926. Many people, often miners and steelworkers, were out of work and eager for a job even if it meant moving south.

Though the First World War had been over for some ten years, many Victorian attitudes persisted in the hospital. The absolute authority of the medical superintendent went unquestioned. The long hours of work (an average 66-hour week for an attendant) and the obsessive division of the sexes for both staff and patients made life austere. A suggestion by the Mental Hospitals Association that it might be possible, on occasions, for female staff to look after male patients, was strongly disapproved of by the Visiting Committee, who attempted to justify their extreme antipathy by reasoning that there was already a difficulty in obtaining female staff and if they had to nurse male patients it would necessitate hiring only those with qualifications for general nursing, thus restricting the pool of potential staff even further.[6]

In their reports of 1932, 1933 and 1934, the Board of Control pointed out that the Homestead was entirely inadequate to the needs of the nursing staff because it only offered accommodation for 22 women. The Committee proposed modest extensions but these were rejected by the Board as unsuitable and unworkable. Eventually, the Visiting Committee appointed a sub-committee to identify a suitable site for the construction of a new nurses' home. The site they chose was a field north of the chapel and behind the medical superintendent's garden.[7]

The builders were Thackeray and Co of Huntingdon, who estimated that the whole building could be erected for a tender price of £21,940.[8] It was opened on 26 July 1937 and undoubtedly improved living conditions for the nursing staff. The Visiting Committee were pleased to note that it also led to a marked decrease in resignations by female staff.

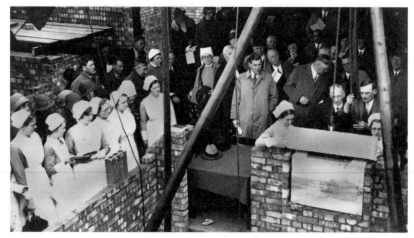

Figure 4.2 Laying the foundation stone for the Nurses' Home, 1937

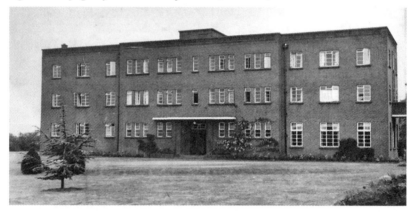

Figure 4.3 Nurses' Home, 1937

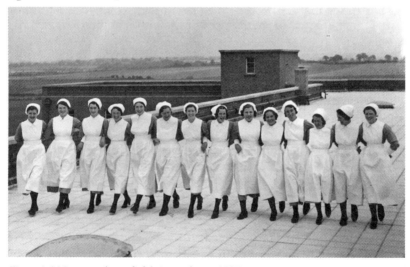

Figure 4.4 Nurses on the roof of their new home, 1937

Fuller died on 15 March 1935, after serving 25 years as medical superintendent. He was succeeded by Dr Neil McDiarmid who had been deputy medical superintendent at the County Mental Hospital, Whittingham, Lancashire.

New Treatments

Following the 1930 Mental Treatment Act, outpatient clinics were set up by the hospital in the towns which fell within the three counties: at Hitchin, Bedford, Luton and Huntingdon. These outpatient clinics were the first tentative steps towards community care. It was thought that treating people while they lived at home might reduce the rate of recurrent admissions. With this initiative in outreach work and a new treatment – insulin coma therapy – becoming established, the medical profession felt more confident than it had for 50 years that they finally had some effective tools to help the increasing numbers of people suffering from mental illness. This period also saw the appearance of other treatments, including the development of occupational therapy.[9] In the mid-1930s a small group of TCH staff began informal training in occupational therapy at other hospitals where this form of therapy had already been instituted.

It is salutary to note that, as late as 1938, Three Counties was still admitting children aged six, seven and eight years old. These were almost exclusively children who had learning difficulties and who should properly have been transferred to the new Bedfordshire and Northamptonshire facility at Bromham, Bedfordshire. In spite of the Mental Deficiency Act of 1913, which legislated a separate category for 'mental defectives', little differentiation was made in practice between those who suffered from mental illness and those who had learning difficulties. They were all treated together at Three Counties, often on the same ward. The Commissioners in Lunacy and, later, the Board of Control often commented on the inadvisability of mixing patient groups, but the pressure of numbers and the shortage of beds meant that it was almost impossible to prevent. The Bromham Hospital opened in 1931, but as it also served the large county of Northamptonshire, it was always full and it wasn't until it was expanded in 1938 that all patients with learning difficulties, including the children, could be transferred.[10]

Insulin coma therapy was used throughout the war years. Not surprisingly, there were dangers associated with putting patients into a coma for an extended period, and a new form of insulin therapy which produced a much shorter period of coma, modified insulin therapy, replaced it. In 1944 insulin therapy was joined by the new electro-convulsive therapy (ECT). Before there were effective major tranquillisers for schizophrenia and severe depression, it was found in

1938 that the use of a brief pulse of electricity of about 800 milliamperes passed across the temple was enough to cause a seizure. The therapy was pioneered by an Italian neuropsychiatrist, Ugo Cerletti, and was taken up around the world as a treatment for serious mental-health problems of all kinds. Cerletti had in fact based his work on the commonly accepted notion that epilepsy and psychosis were mutually exclusive, that is to say if you were epileptic then you were unlikely to have a severe psychotic disorder. This is in fact untrue, subsequent research has shown, but at the time this idea led researchers to look for effective ways of inducing epileptic convulsions and Cerletti's electrical method was by far the easiest way to do this. ECT still has a place in modern psychiatry as it has been shown to be effective in cases of severe depression and in some bipolar conditions where medication does not provide relief. Dr Robert Russell, who came to work at Three Counties just before the war and returned in 1946, recalls the excitement generated amongst the staff by these new approaches during this period:

> The techniques [ECT] came to Britain in 1939 and we had our first machine when I came back to Three Counties after the war. It was made by Ediswan and it wasn't much use. It was early days and no-one knew the ideal size or duration of shock to induce a useful convulsion. I did some experiments and found that the Ediswan machine could not really give enough volts so I went back to my rooms at the Three Counties and built my own machine. I was an electronics hobbyist so I thought I would make something that worked better than the commercial machine.
>
> We used it for both depression and severe psychosis. It produced wonderful results. We worked at it until it was right and I thought that for depressives and some intransigent schizophrenics, it was unbeatable. It was so quick and you didn't have to be in hospital to receive treatment. We had an ECT suite in the new admission block (the Fairfield Unit) and people would come on an outpatient basis two or three times a week for a course of treatment. They would arrive in the morning then go home in the afternoon. Within a week most of them were better.[11] That was something unique to Three Counties and it was very popular.
>
> The short coma induced by insulin was not terribly useful, we discovered. It was good for building up patients with poor appetites but by 1947 we had pretty much stopped using it and had gone over to ECT. We also tried fever therapy. A high fever was felt to be useful for those with neurosyphilis and we occasionally used this technique. We would receive malarial mosquitoes from the Maudsley

Hospital and we had to be careful to ensure the mosquitoes only bit the patient! We didn't use it much and gave it up altogether by 1949. Penicillin had come in and it was much more useful.[12]

Following the 1930 Mental Treatment Act, it was also necessary to upgrade the facilities on the Three Counties site and in 1936 it was proposed that a new admission block be built to receive only voluntary patients. Parrott and Dunham, the Luton Borough architects, were commissioned to come up with plans for a new unit to be situated in an area between the main building and Wilbury Farm. It consisted of a male and female ward, each with twenty beds, plus specialist rooms for hydrotherapy and insulin therapy and a small operating theatre. It was opened by the Chairman of the Board of Control for Lunacy and Mental Deficiency Sir Laurence Brock on 26 June 1939 as 'Fairfield Hospital' but was almost immediately requisitioned by the war department for use as a ward for officer casualties and as part of the Emergency Hospital Scheme. Two stand-alone villa wards were built on either side for sixteen patients each and designated as 'convalescent units' for rehabilitating recovering patients.

The War Years and the Immediate Post-War Period

The Second World War and the immediate post-war period ushered in great changes for the hospital. Between 1938 and 1940 new buildings were constructed, including the (female) nurses' home, admission block, villas and the hutted Emergency Hospital. The expansion led to a period of intense activity in what had previously been a rather isolated institution.

With the prospect of war, it was realised that the London hospitals would be prone to bombing and the authorities looked around for rural locations where patients could be safely treated. Provincial mental hospitals like the Three Counties were already full and it was planned that a large contingent of patients be moved out to create space. In March 1939, five months before the outbreak of hostilities, the Emergency Hospital Scheme had been initiated by the Ministry of Health and two consultants had, at the behest of the government, come up from London to arrange how best to accommodate parts of the Royal Free Hospital on site. By August, 147 Three Counties patients had been evacuated to Fulbourn in Cambridgeshire and 200 to Northampton, mostly Huntingdon patients plus some from Bedford Borough. Although the transfer was meant as a temporary measure – 'for the duration of the present National Emergency' – it became a permanent arrangement, at least for the Huntingdon patients.[13] Thus ended an association between the Three Counties Hospital and the

County of Huntingdonshire which had lasted some 79 years. The 347 beds released by the move were used for patients from Hill End Hospital in St Albans, whose catchment area included south Hertfordshire and North London. Hill End itself was used to accommodate staff and patients from St Bartholomew's, the London teaching hospital.

The war years also exacerbated a problem that Three Counties had been struggling with for at least twenty years: the shortage of both male and female nursing staff. Throughout the 1939–45 period difficulties in recruitment had to be countered by rising wages in an attempt to match the pay that was on offer from local factories engaged in war work. Initially, this was rather modest but it was subject to regular review, and by 1945 typical weekly wages had risen from £2 13s for a nurse in 1939 to £4 2s.[14] Despite all efforts, the numbers of female nurses in particular began to drop to desperate levels. In their 1941 report, the Commissioners of the Board of Control highlighted the difficulty:

> The shortage of nursing staff, particularly on the female side, is serious and the staff of women nurses is nearly one-third below strength. In consequence one or two wards are undoubtedly understaffed notably on Ward Female 4 [the refractory ward for female patients who were slow to recover], where there are at present only four nurses for 83 patients, nine of whom are a 'suicide risk'. We mention this only to emphasise the difficulties under which the Hospital is working and not, unfortunately, because we are able to suggest a means of solving them.[15]

The medical superintendent, Neil McDiarmid, even wrote to the Board of Control in February 1942 suggesting that female national service women should be drafted to work at the hospital, adding, 'this will have to be done later on but it should be done now – before serious accidents occur'.[16] As numbers continued to fall, the Visiting Committee petitioned the Regional Controller of the Ministry of Labour in December 1944 and was allowed to advertise in the Belfast and Dublin newspapers for student and assistant nurses.[17] This produced twenty replies and a number of these came to Three Counties as students in June 1944. Ireland was to become a major recruiting area for the hospital for the next forty years.

Staff shortages also affected the medical staff, and by 1942 two senior medical assistants, Drs Page and Russell, had been called up. McDiarmid was not only in charge of Three Counties but also acted as the head of the busy Emergency Hospital on site. Dr Finieffs remained in post as deputy medical superintendent, and Dr Menzies (who dealt mainly with physical ailments) as the solitary senior medical assistant. Finieffs continued using insulin coma therapy during the war years and, in 1944, brought in the first electro-convulsing machine. The University of London applied to have Three Counties Hospital recognised as a centre for training medical students on the mental-health course because of the 'modern methods of treatment used'.[18] Thereafter, students regularly came to the hospital for placement during training and received lectures from McDiarmid and Finieffs.

Because of its rural location, there was little likelihood of Three Counties Hospital being bombed, but it could certainly act as a beacon for enemy bombers and was subject to the same blackout and other restrictions that affected the rest of the population. As well as the Emergency Hospital that was being hastily erected near to the path that connected the 'Big House' (as the main building was called locally) to the new admissions block, a searchlight unit was established at Wilbury Farm.[19]

On 15 March 1941 a number of incendiary bombs were dropped by enemy aircraft onto the farm buildings at Wilbury; the bombers were probably returning from a raid and were off-loading. It seems little damage was done apart from a few holes in the roof. Two farm workers were first on the scene and, due to their prompt action, only one haystack was lost.[20]

Towards the end of the war, in March 1945, the hospital took on its first psychologist, who split her duties between Three Counties Asylum and the Bromham Hospital.[21] Another more radical form of treatment began around this time as well. McDiarmid explained to his colleagues that there was excitement over a brain operation called a 'pre-frontal lobotomy', which was thought to be effective, particularly where there were intractable symptoms of schizophrenia with strong delusional and aggressive components. This operation was radical because it severed the connections in the brain to the pre-frontal areas which were thought to control brain activity.[22] The procedure was taken up enthusiastically from the 1940s until the mid-1950s, when it gave way to the new drug-based therapies. W. McKissock of Kings College Hospital, London, began to perform pre-frontal lobotomies at Three Counties in July 1943.[23]

The following case history from this era illustrates some of the effects of pre-frontal lobotomy on patients. G.W., aged 28, was admitted to TCH in December 1943 from a military hospital and was diagnosed as suffering from schizophrenia. He was described as 'childish' and 'irresponsible'. He persistently pestered female visitors and suffered from 'voices in his head dictating his actions'. He had been an army driver in the Middle East who had his first breakdown during action in the desert. The War Office accepted that G. W.'s condition was 'aggravated by', but, they argued, 'not attributable to, his war Service'. His day-to-day activity level was low and he was consistently described as 'apathetic' and 'lacking any emotion' although there were instances of unpredictable aggressive outbursts.

He was first treated with insulin coma therapy and ECT but appeared to derive no lasting improvement from either. In 1945 he was given a pre-frontal lobotomy by McKissock. He was considered recovered enough two days later to return to his ward, but was kept under special observation. For the first week, it is noted that he was 'somnolent and dreamy' but otherwise not complaining of discomfort. However, within a fortnight he had become aggressive and the nurses noted that 'he is lashing out and giving us much trouble which required sedation'. He quietened within a week but began to have a number of epileptic fits which were thought to have been caused by the operation. Despite this, he was given home leave for short periods while in hospital and the fits gradually ceased. He was discharged soon after and was followed up by a home visit from the psychiatric social worker some three months later, who wrote 'the patient is very cheerful and hard working. His father says G. W. changed after the operation. Before, he was very smart, attaching great importance to his clothes and appearance. Afterwards he had a tendency to neglect himself, but had "no worries".' His case was closed some six months after the operation with a notation of 'Total Recovery'.[24]

Outcomes of lobotomy varied considerably. A medical textbook of the period cautions that, 'It is probable that every individual after the operation is happier than before but this may be bought at too great a cost.'[25] Much of a patient's selfhood was given up with the loss of part of the frontal lobe, which produced what was called 'defrontalised dementia'.[26] While the treatment undoubtedly helped some it also led in other cases to very disabled and agitated patients. The procedure was controversial for a range of reasons: it was a serious operation that could not be reversed, it cut connections to the higher functions of the brain with unpredictable results and it caused no little ethical discomfort within the profession. In any event, with new and effective pharmaceutical products coming onto the market the procedure was quietly abandoned during the early 1950s.

The Post-War Period

As the Second World War drew to a close, the medical superintendent wrote to the War Ministry requesting the return of the admission block then known as Fairfield Hospital. He was told that in the light of the continuing hostilities against Japan, it could not be relinquished since it was still needed to treat officers.[27] By October of that year the war was over and the searchlight unit at Wilbury Farm was dismantled and sold as scrap. A circular was sent to all hospitals from the Board of Control containing a letter of thanks to all hospital workers from both Houses of Parliament.[28] The National Health Service Act of 1946 brought TCH into the North West Thames Health Region and McDiarmid was appointed to a special task force to look at where to place outpatient clinics for mental-health patients throughout the new region.[29] The coming of the NHS in 1948 swept away the autonomous mental hospitals and placed them into a structure which sought to ensure uniformity of treatments and patient care and of staff working conditions and training. This move to greater standardisation was regretted by some of the medical officers, as the friendly rivalry between hospitals had brought about some progressive innovations during the inter-war years. From then on all experimentation would have to be subjected to the scrutiny of the NHS.

The NHS management also stipulated that all nursing staff should be properly qualified so that the mental-health service would be on a par with general hospitals. Although there had been a policy in place for twenty years at TCH of encouraging staff to take recognised exams and certificates, it had never been mandatory. However, the new scale of wages for nurses dictated that all unqualified staff had to be re-classified as nursing assistants, in spite of their achieved status within the hospital's own nursing hierarchy. Many male and female nurses with long service records found themselves classed as nursing assistants on a lower salary scale than their colleagues who had taken a qualification. Due to the shortage of staff, the medical superintendent advised the Visiting Committee to pay such staff the top wages allowable, in order to retain their services and in respect of their great experience.[30]

In October 1946 parts of the admission block were vacated by the Royal Free and were at last partially re-opened to psychiatric patients.[31] The insulin and ECT suites were re-situated there from the Homestead and TCH went on to be recognised as a centre of expertise for these treatments. By the end of 1946, teaching programmes had been instituted at TCH for psychiatrists from other hospitals.[32]

With the end of the war, the Emergency Hospital could be dismantled and in early 1947 a number of staff were made redundant, while the Ministry of Health considered what to do with the huts. It had signed a 25-year lease with TCH in 1939 and this still had some seventeen years to run. The Visiting Committee was informed that the London Chest Hospital would take up residence in late 1947 as they needed a countryside location which would suit convalescent patients.[33] There had been some detailed negotiation as to how this new hospital within the grounds of the Three Counties would be serviced. It had, after all, its own staff and was an entirely separate organisation and yet required all the food, washing and cleaning facilities that any large hospital needed. It was decided that the contract which had existed with the Royal Free Hospital during the war should continue, which meant, in essence, that all electricity, water and provisioning would come through the TCH system. Laundry, however, was a more contentious issue. The bedding and clothing from the London Chest was likely to be heavily contaminated with tuberculosis and would require a dedicated laundry to prevent cross infection. All large institutions feared epidemics and the TCH had had a great deal of experience of diphtheria, typhoid, paratyphoid, dysentery and tuberculosis over the 87 years it had been open. The Visiting Committee decided in the end that the London Chest would have to make its own laundering arrangements.

By November 1947 the Fairfield admission block was at last fully re-opened to voluntary patients. It had been handed back to the TCH some months earlier but lack of male staff had delayed its formal opening.[34]

The role of psychiatric social workers (known as PSWs) was discussed in a meeting of the Visiting Committee in January 1948 when one of the members asked whether adequate aftercare arrangements were in place for discharged patients.[35] Surprisingly, the term 'aftercare' was in use during this period, meaning substantially what it does today: the follow-up care and support offered to people discharged from hospital and living in the community. The question had been raised on this occasion because two former patients of TCH had committed suicide while at home. The report gives a flavour of what aftercare meant in 1948:

> The Medical Superintendent explained that in both cases the relatives had been advised to return the patients to hospital for further treatment but had not done so. In reply to the question – Dr McDiarmid re-assured the Visiting Committee that there were 2 PSWs employed to visit and report on patients discharged from Three Counties Hospital.

In December 1947 the Visiting Committee agreed that the Homestead, now empty again after the opening of the admission block, should be converted into a Nurse Training School with some room set aside for flats. At almost the same time the first students were being taken on for a three-year course for the Registered Mental Nursing (RMN) qualification. This new national qualification was a great improvement on the probationer nurse scheme of the 1930s: it had a government-

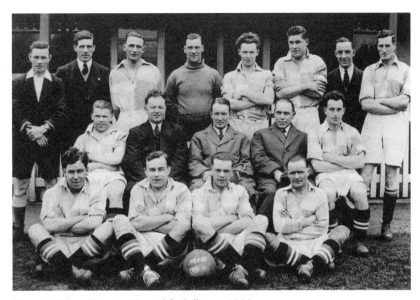

Figure 4.5 Three Counties Hospital football team, 1933

approved curriculum with a structured and monitored range of placements so that the trainees could build up a diversity of skills.

Students were expected to attend for work before school started at 9.30am during the week. The hours for nursing staff were long: 7.00am–7.00pm six days per week. Because of nursing shortages, Three Counties Hospital paid an enhanced rate to nursing students and other staff and consequently enjoyed a reputation for being a good employer. At the labour exchange in Arlesey it was common knowledge that though they advertised for staff for both Arlesey Brick Co. and Three Counties, to get into the latter you either had to play cricket or a musical instrument. Certainly, the cricket team made up of members of staff had played a prominent part in the history of the Hospital and during the 1920s and 1930s in particular was recognised as a county-level team.

It's clear that, at this time, while staff and patients occupied essentially the same space – the hospital, the grounds and so forth – they represented two very different cultures. All the significant social events – the dances, the cricket team, the band and the gala – were designed principally to entertain staff and their guests. The patients on the other hand had their activities arranged for them and during the 1940s and early 1950s they had what looked like a busy week:

Monday   Country dancing
Tuesday   Film show/Dancing

Wednesday	Visitors' night
Thursday	Craft
Friday	Dance night
Saturday	Concert or show given by local societies

But change was in the air. The traditions of the large mental hospitals which seemed so immutable were being challenged by the sweeping innovations to British society that the post-War Atlee government brought into being. The creation of the Welfare State included the founding of a National Health Service which was entirely free at the point of use for every citizen. The new NHS took on virtually all the existing general and mental hospitals around the country and they immediately made it clear they intended to follow government policy as announced in a White Paper in 1944[36] – to close the existing large hospital sites and instead transfer mental-health care to the aegis of the local general hospitals.

In August 1947 the Visiting Committee were notified by the Region that they should wind up their affairs by July 1948. With the transfer of authority for mental hospitals from the county councils to central government, it had been decided that new Management Committees should take over from the long-established Committees of Visitors. At the last meeting of the Visiting Committee on 8 June 1948, it was also reported that the new North West Thames Regional Health Authority had fixed the catchment area for TCH as 'the whole of Bedfordshire and North Hertfordshire as from 5 July 1948'.[37] In fact, virtually all the same people from the Visiting Committee sat on the new Management Committee when it took up responsibility for overseeing the running of the hospital on 10 June 1948.

In December 1948, Dr Colman Kenton reported to the Management Committee that, in future, the medical staff at the hospital would be increased to ten doctors: two consultants (including the medical superintendent), two assistant psychiatrists, two senior registrars, two junior registrars and two other medical officers. Given that they had just struggled through the war years with four medical staff, this must have appeared to be a generous allotment.[38]

The NHS retained the Board of Control, but in future they were to report directly to the Minister for Health. The twice-yearly visits to review the facilities and monitor patient care by the re-formed Board of Control continued and on 30 May 1949 they commented on the upgrading work being undertaken at the hospital.[39] They noted that the nurse training school was now ready to open its doors. Many of the new medical posts had been filled too. The new roster now consisted of:

Consultants	Dr Neil McDiarmid, Dr L Page
Senior Registrars	Dr D McDowell, Dr F Shattock
Registrars	Dr J Glynn, Dr B Campden Main
Senior Hospital Officer	Dr R Russell
Junior Hospital Officer	Dr E Menzies

A new hospital chaplain, the Rev. A.S. Monk from Henlow Parish, was also appointed in January 1950.[40] The chaplaincy, the house halfway down the Arlesey Drive, had by this time been divided into two flats. A social worker lived in one with her mother, and Rev. Monk was given the other and took up residence on 1 May 1950.

Creating a Modern Psychiatric Service 1950–60

Since the war, the new Management Committee had vacillated about finding new male staff accommodation. Many of the officers of the hospital (i.e. the medical staff, the senior administrator and the heads of departments) lived in houses in the hospital grounds, as did many of the farming staff. Yet few, if any, male nurses were so lucky. Like their Victorian predecessors, many of them were still occupying the side rooms off the wards in the main building. This arrangement was extremely unpopular and was affecting recruitment.

In February 1950 Henlow Grange, a large house in nearby Henlow village, was put up for lease and a deputation from the Management Committee examined it to see if it could be usefully made into a new male nursing home.[41] Finding it too far away and too expensive (at £250 per year) for the hospital's needs, they declined. In October a large house by the war memorial in Arlesey village came up for sale – Arlesey Bury. The Management Committee sought permission to put in a bid and the place was acquired from ITC (International Computers and Tabulators) who were based in Letchworth. In spite of the fact that the building was very dilapidated, staff were housed there immediately. The garden was growing wild, the swimming pool cracked and empty and the conservatory unusable. Two or three beds were put in each of the large rooms with little or no refurbishment. The nursing staff, far from appearing grateful, complained. The Management Committee were nonplussed and responded:

> We cannot agree that the accommodation is unsatisfactory. Previously resident Male Nurses were only accommodated in rooms adjacent to the Wards where they were liable to be disturbed by patients and where they had little privacy. As permission to build a new Home has not been granted, the only solution has been to look for accommodation outside. In a recent report, the Board of Control stated 'Arlesey Bury

is the finest of its kind that we have seen – many Hospitals in London have nursing staff accommodated several miles from their place of work'. We even provide transport to and from Arlesey Bury and apart from the issue of central heating [i.e. there were fireplaces but no central heating] we feel that it is entirely adequate.[42]

Within a few years, at the behest of the Board of Control, the exterior was painted but the interior remained untouched. After a second visit, the Board of Control observed:

> We thought [Arlesey Bury] greatly in need of decoration and understood that it was to be done soon. We deprecate the fact that there are 3 or 4 beds in some rooms but realise that the size of the rooms makes this inevitable. Peeling walls and chipped paint make parts of the house dreary. Redecoration with some other improvements would make a difference. The grounds ... give the impression of being derelict and the glass houses have suffered much at the hands of hooligans. A fence should be erected around the building as it seems it is far too accessible to passers-by.[43]

Arlesey Bury was to remain the main male nursing quarters until 1965 when much of the hutted area was vacated by the London Chest Hospital staff. The Bury was then sold to a member of Arlesey Parish Council and stood empty for some years before being demolished to make way for the Chase Farm housing estate in the early 1970s.

It is interesting to note that the strict separation of the sexes insisted on in Victorian times continued throughout the 1950s and on into the 'permissive' 1960s, when checks were still being made on the female nurses' residences at night to ensure there were no men on site. The integration of the nurses' home had to wait until 1979. The old order was gradually giving way, but TCH and other large hospitals retained their traditional practices far longer than many other sectors of society. This was probably partly due to institutional inertia, but also to their very self-sufficiency which meant that there was little need to update their practices in order to attract new staff. Things were changing incrementally and while society moved to adapt to new ideas and imperatives, the lives within the closed confines of the institution were forced to move forward too, albeit at a slower rate.

The number of patients in the hospital remained very high and the level rarely fell below 1,200, with even more coming in on a daily basis to occupational therapy or to work on the land or in the laundry. The vast majority of in-patients spent only a short time in hospital and frequently came in voluntarily under the 1930 Mental Health

Treatment Act. Of the 830 admissions in 1951, 763 departed within the year.

The number of medical officers stayed doggedly at eight despite the longstanding recommendation from the Region that ten posts should be filled. A Senior Registrar, F. Shattock, ran a clinical research unit based in the Fairfield Hospital block. She and her team of two scientists (an endocrinologist and a chemist) produced a number of learned papers regarding the biochemical bases of mental illness.[44] Russell's work on ECT also attracted a great deal of interest. The outpatient clinics in Bedford and at Luton and Dunstable Hospitals were very busy and the Nurse Training School was full with 39 students – 'the majority being French girls'.[45]

To mark the coronation of Queen Elizabeth II in June 1953, the hospital planned a week of celebrations. A large-screen Decca television was purchased for £185 and the chaplain arranged a programme of events.[46] The patients were allowed to watch the ceremony in relays during the day and evening on the television which had been set up in the female hall. A patients' 'Coronation Dance' was held on Wednesday 3 June, a concert by the hospital orchestra on Thursday and on Friday there was a large Coronation Ball for staff and guests.

Unfortunately, Daniel McDowell, one of the senior registrars, died suddenly on his way to the Friday ball and the festivities were cut short. A report written later by Rev. Monk tells the story:

> The Hospital suffered a grievous loss during Coronation Week: all had gone excellently until just after 9.00 pm on the night of the Staff Ball. Dr McDowell left the Hospital Lodge [at the rear of the Hospital in those days] saying that he was going to fetch Mrs McDowell; five minutes afterwards he was found lying on the Church Hill. He was brought back to the hospital by Dr Page and Dr Russell and they, together with the Medical Superintendent, fought for some hours to see if they could revive him but he had passed beyond all human aid. Immediately it became known, the Staff Ball was abandoned.[47]

The New Year's Eve Ball

Dances at the hospital, which, it's worth noting, were solely for staff and their guests, had become substantial affairs by this time. TCH was famous locally and farther afield for the lavishness of its events and, particularly, the quality of the food. Emerging from rationing, the country was beginning to regain its taste for enjoying life. Before the war, the New Year's Eve Ball had been the major event of the local social calendar but it had not been held during the war. With the availability of farm produce, it was possible after the war to provide occasional feasts 'off-ration' for big parties such as the New Year's Eve and Halloween Balls. The Police also started to book the hospital for Midsummer Balls and they also became a regular event.

Reg Buck, who was for many years the catering manager at the hospital, recalls those days:

> I came to work at TCH after the war in 1946 when I came out of the Army. I was stationed at Arlesey and married a local girl so I thought I would settle here. I had my interview with Dr McDiarmid and Mr Whalley, the hospital secretary. The hospital band was smashing then. There was Jack Batey on piano, Sid Pearce on drums and Freddie Gibbs played the saxophone. Mr Warburton was the kitchen superintendent and he was responsible for planning the menus for the big dances, ordering food and its preparation. It was like a military campaign and we started planning for the New Year's Eve Ball in September. The centrepiece was a pig's head but there were hams and other meats – all things that were difficult to get at the time.[48]

Margaret Moore, who came to TCH in 1948 and was one of the first students through the Preliminary Nursing School, also recalled the large dances:

> You had real status working at the Three Counties – especially at New Year's or Halloween – because of the balls that were organised. Tickets were like gold dust and everyone who was anyone wanted to be there. The dance was held in the female hall and the band was really quite famous – all of them were hospital staff. I remember Freddie Gibbs on sax and Vernon Hall who played the violin. He also played the chapel organ on Sunday.[49]

Possible Expansion

In July 1952 the gasworks at the top of the Arlesey Drive, near to the Orchard, was demolished. It had for many years been in a parlous and probably dangerous state. At the same time, the tramway was deemed unnecessary, since its main purpose had been to bring coal to the gasworks. Stutley Bros of Stevenage were awarded the contract and were allowed, in part payment, to sell the metal rails and sleepers for scrap. The cost of this operation was £2,500, which included filling in the cuttings, making good the roads and fitting kerbing along the Arlesey Drive. It was rumoured that an old carriage had been jammed under the bridge to speed filling in the cutting but there is no record of this. All the work was completed by March 1953.[50] The weighbridge was still required and was left in place, near to the barrier on the way to the old hospital boilerhouse. Both the tramway and the gasworks had been built before the main building and so had been in existence some 95 years.

During 1953, the London Chest Hospital began to hand back a number of hutted wards to TCH because of low bed occupancy. With the NHS now firmly established, this was timely. Over the years it had become clear that the geriatric patient population within the Three Counties was growing and it was envisaged that this age group would form a sizeable contingent within a few years. Until the 1950s, the elderly had been cared for on wards with the general mix of patients, despite their particular needs. Several Board of Control Reports from 1948 onwards had commented on the need for specialist geriatric accommodation, and the huts were quickly refurbished and pressed into use. As the London Chest retreated from the site over the next ten years, the huts would come to play a significant role and remain in use until the closure of the hospital in 1999.

In September 1953 a working party from the Regional Board examined TCH and concluded that perhaps it was time to consider building a new mental hospital altogether and they suggested that it should be in Stevenage.[51] McDiarmid assured the Board that this was not necessary, if only money could be found to upgrade the existing site. He claimed that the provision of new buildings and the upgrading of the main hospital would, even by the most pessimistic predictions, be undertaken within the next ten or twenty years.

In the event, the psychiatric unit at Stevenage would have to wait another fifteen years to be built and the Board instead recommended that TCH should be upgraded as follows:

- more accommodation for female patients
- houses for married doctors
- a new x-ray machine
- complete re-wiring of the main building
- new toilets throughout the hospital
- new dining facilities for male staff[52]

Televisions were appearing in the wards and a large-screen, rear-projection TV was purchased for £245 for the Male Hall for those not lucky enough to have one in their area.

Changes in Philosophy

The number of patients under the care of the medical and nursing staff remained at a high level through the 1950s but it is interesting to note that they were being treated under two different pieces of legislation.

Clearly, the intention of the 1930 Mental Treatment Act had been to gradually replace the 1890 Lunacy Act, which only allowed for 'certified' detention. It was hoped in 1930 that ten or twenty years down the line (i.e., by 1950), the vast majority of patients would be 'voluntary' rather than certified. In June 1954, the numbers were as follows:[53]

Males		Females		Totals		Grand
Certified	Voluntary	Certified	Voluntary	Certified	Voluntary	Total
342	182	482	204	824	386	1210
(524)		(686)				

Patient numbers in 1954[54]

Twenty-four years after the 1930 Act, only 34% of male patients and 30% of female patients were voluntary. This is not quite as damning as it might appear: 85% of all *new* admissions came in voluntarily under the 1930 Act, but that did leave 15% being admitted as certified patients under the 1890 Act.

Before 1948, general and psychiatric hospitals had developed quite separately and were run in completely different ways. The coming of the NHS brought them together under the same overall management for the first time. The physical upgrading of the old asylums was deemed the first priority, since their standards – on the whole – were well below those acceptable to general hospitals. Yet there was only so much that could be done to the massive Victorian buildings to bring them up to standard. TCH, like other large hospitals up and down the country, was finding it difficult, due to a lack of resources, to meet the expectations of the new Board of Control to radically upgrade as a matter of urgency.

The Board of Control's figures show that in 1954 some 151,400 people were cared for in large asylums across the country, representing over 30% of the total hospital population, yet the proportion of money spent by the NHS on the mental-health services was only 16%. A parliamentary debate in February 1954[55] citing these figures was notable because it was to lead, some five years later, to a radical change in mental-health law. It drew attention to four major deficiencies in the mental-health services: a shortage of beds, suitable buildings, staff and money.

The public attention generated by the debate led, between 1954 and 1959, to a revolution in patient care. In fact, there were three revolutions – a pharmacological one, a social one and, finally, with the passing of the 1959 Mental Health Act, a legislative one. The pharmacological revolution came with the development of psychotropic medication such as tranquillisers, sedatives and anti-depressants. The most notable new drug was chlorpromazine, which had a powerful anti-psychotic effect and started to become available from 1954. In TCH, as in all large hospitals, patients were responding to these new medications and the result was a far quieter and more settled atmosphere. Many patients were able to return home. The new drugs were not a cure for severe mental illness, but they did alleviate many of the distressing symptoms and gave a greater level of control to the patients themselves. Drug therapy also meant that it was possible to think about alternative ways of caring for the mentally ill. For Victorian institutions, which, despite the enlightened intentions of their designers, had come to represent an unacceptable face of mental-health care, drug therapy was ultimately to signal the beginning of their demise.

Maxwell Jones, a South-African-born psychiatrist working at Mill Hill Hospital in North London, was developing at this time what came to be known as the 'therapeutic community'.[56] The formal lines of communication between mental-health professionals and their patients were replaced by a more egalitarian regime where the running of the unit was conducted through group meetings. At many psychiatric units, day hospitals were established where patients could live at home and attend clinics and therapy sessions on an out-patient basis. This was a radical new way of working and was termed the 'open-door system'. These images of modern mental-health care were to feature highly in the process of drafting the new mental-health legislation.

Three Counties Hospital attempted to keep up with some of the changes. The Board of Control Report for October 1954 records the efforts that were being made:

> The improvements effected on the wards are really astonishing and Dr McDiarmid, the Medical Superintendent and Mr Whaley, the Secretary are to be warmly congratulated. All the wards in the main building have been re-decorated in light and pleasing colours, there is fluorescent lighting and curtains in every ward. The difference after the last 2 years is truly remarkable ... Everywhere there is a good supply of flowers.[57]

The Board of Control Commissioner noted in his tour around the grounds that:

> The Hospital is geographically remote from centres of population and residences are urgently required for at least 4 Medical Officers. For the same reason, a well-equipped staff canteen and Social Club (with a club licence) would help recruitment and induce existing staff to remain.

This view was supported by the Regional Hospital Board when it considered how to develop services in the Hertfordshire and Bedfordshire area. It concluded that the following upgrades to TCH were urgently required:[58]

- 200 more beds for female patients
- 4 new houses for doctors' residences
- New dining room for staff

Some £3000 was made available by the Region, but this was nowhere near enough to deal with the overcrowding which was their priority problem. A partial solution was to come along at the end of 1954 when the London Chest Hospital was able to hand over two more huts, and these were adapted and upgraded for mental-health patients.

By 1955, despite its attempts at modernisation, the hospital maintained a traditional approach to patient care and overcrowding was still a problem. For example, 63 patients had been boarded out since the war at St Crispin's Hospital in Northampton and there was little likelihood of them returning. Although the Fairfield Unit, the Nurse Training School and the doctors' training programmes were all achievements compared to many of the large hospitals at the time, there were still definite deficiencies.

End of the Asylum Era

In 1954 the Regional Board decided that all farming activity in the hospitals should cease. In response to this, Three Counties had done little more than move the cattle and other livestock to Wilbury Farm and close the old Three Counties farmyard. Farm work and gardening were at this time still the main daytime activities undertaken by male patients. Overall the hospital had the use of some 406 acres of land (about 165 hectares), most of it owned by the hospital but some leased from local farmers. The Minister of Health sent a letter to each hospital asking for proposals to wind up all existing farming activity as soon as possible.[59] The Region advised:

> That an area of some 198 acres should be retained at Three Counties Hospital, this area comprising the 101 acres of land on which the hospital buildings stand and the 97 acres at present farmed as arable land. This would involve the termination of the lease at present held in respect of the 92 acres and the disposal by sale of the 116 acres of grassland. Of the land to be retained the Sub-Committee propose that the existing 97 acres of arable land should be leased, subject to suitable restrictions and rights being arranged.[60]

This meant the hospital would be allowed to lease the remaining farmland to others but not farm it themselves. The Committee were clearly taken aback at the scale of the cutback that the Region demanded – after all, TCH had been involved in farming since 1858. They wrote back saying that these proposals were entirely unacceptable and requesting a meeting with the Health Minister but, in the end, the NHS managers proved unyielding. In March 1956 the Committee had no choice but to give instructions to the farm manager to sell all his livestock over the summer and it was agreed that Wilbury Farm would be put up for auction in September. Despite the cutbacks, there were still about 200 acres attached to the hospital and many of the staff continued to live on the site either in the Nurses' home or in the number of cottages that were traditionally reserved for senior staff in the hospital grounds.

In 1956 McDiarmid announced his retirement and was warmly praised by both the Board of Control and the Management Committee for his work. Fred Crouch, the hospital's chief engineer, had also retired some months earlier, in December 1955. Fred had been at the hospital throughout the installation of the electricity in the 1920s and had also taken on the massive job of fitting central heating throughout the main building. Coal fires on each ward were still a feature of hospital life at this time, but in the early 1950s moves had been made to fit electric heaters in some of the wards. This had proved too expensive and in

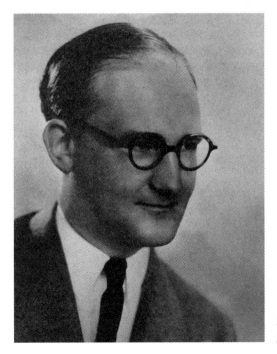

Figure 4.6 Leslie Ford,
Medical Superintendent, c. 1950

1954 it was decided to provide hot–water central heating to each ward. It was a massive undertaking and Crouch regretted that he had not completed the task before he retired.[61] J. Harahan, who was chief engineer at Sheffield Mental Hospital, was appointed as his successor.

The new medical superintendent, Dr Leslie Ford, took up his post on 1 June 1956. One of the first changes initiated by Ford was the move to the three-shift system for nurses in November 1956. This was recommended by the Region and was adopted by both general and mental hospitals. The London Chest Hospital also made two more wards available to the hospital and these were upgraded and used for elderly patients. The move towards the use of the huts for elderly patients was being put in place and would remain until the closure of the hospital.

Percy Whaley retired as group secretary on 31 May 1957, after 43 years of service. He had worked at the hospital since 1914 and many, indeed most, of those working at Three Counties could not remember a time before his appointment as clerk and steward in 1937. He had proved to be hugely influential over the years, a patrician figure in the hospital hierarchy, whose views were sought by the most senior staff, including the various medical superintendents he had worked under. To honour his legacy the Committee agreed to name his hospital residence after him and put up a small plaque on what came to be known as Whaley House. He was replaced by John Russell, who took up his appointment as group secretary and finance officer in June 1957.[62]

Institutions under Attack

In 1961 the American sociologist Erving Goffman published his influential book *Asylums*, which looked at the culture of what he called 'total institutions' and pointed out the effects of what came to be termed 'institutionalisation' on both staff and residents. According to Goffman, every aspect of life in large institutions subtly reinforced a blinkered loyalty and dependence. The pathology of institutional life, as outlined by Goffman, did not only relate to mental hospitals (although his study had come out of his experiences at St Elizabeth's Mental Hospital in Washington DC where he did ethnographic research) but to prisons, old people's homes, boarding schools and the military. Goffman named practices common in all these insular societies which, while seemingly innocuous, were, he maintained, engendering an unhealthy and debilitating dependence in those affected. Everything about hospital culture was examined and held up as evidence of the detrimental effect of 'total institutional care' from the Sports Day to the rituals associated with New Year's Balls.

He wrote:

> Two different social and cultural worlds develop, jogging alongside
> each other with points of official contact but little mutual penetration.
> Significantly, the institutional plant and name come to be identified
> by both staff and inmates as somehow only belonging to the staff so
> that when anybody refers to the views or interests of the institution,
> they are referring … to the views and concerns of the staff.[63]

Goffman pointed to a patient sub-culture which had its own linguistic code
and thrived on scavenging for food and tobacco, running illegal exchange
systems and avoiding the more onerous duties imposed by staff around
them. Goffman argued that institutional life was essentially abnormal but
that this was only obvious to those on the outside – those within it were
oblivious to the disabling effects of institutionalisation. Goffman's direct
style ensured that the book attracted a wide readership and the assumption
that institutional life was in some way 'normal' was challenged.

The work of Goffman and others was to lead within a very short
time to acceptance, certainly in government at the time, of the idea
that the days of the large residential hospital were numbered. At TCH
things had been moving in this direction in any case – the farm had
been sold off by NHS decree, the powers of the medical superintendent
and the medical staff had been circumscribed by new regulations, and
in 1959 the new Mental Health Act came into force. This legislation
swept in a set of new rights for patients, including the right of consent
and appeal, which allowed patients to challenge medical decisions
and, by extension, the long-held belief in the autocracy of doctors.
Significantly, the role of medical superintendent was also abolished and
Ford's title was changed to consultant psychiatrist.

Under Enoch Powell, the Ministry of Health issued a document
proposing radical changes to mental health policy which was
innocuously titled 'A Hospital Plan for England and Wales'.[64] The
'Hospital Plan' proposed a restriction on hospital services and laid out
the policy that, in future, the mentally ill, the mentally handicapped
and the elderly would no longer occupy hospital beds for long periods.
Psychiatric care was to be concentrated in the district general hospital
which would provide acute treatment in all medical specialist areas. The
intention was that patients would enter hospital only for a short period
for diagnosis and assessment, and their on-going care would be then a
matter for community services. At the formation of the NHS in 1948,
nearly 40% of all hospital beds were psychiatric, and over a fourteen-
year period a great deal of money had been put into upgrading this
neglected sector.[65] As a result, the medical acute services had been to

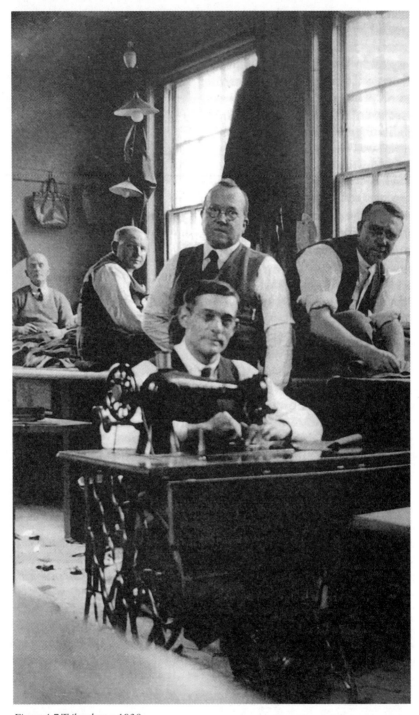

Figure 4.7 Tailor shop, c.1930

some extent neglected and they urgently needed funds to build new district general hospitals.

By 1960, after a century of institutional life at TCH, radical changes to patient care and psychiatric treatment were beginning to be felt. Patient labour was outlawed,[66] the 1959 Act had given patients new rights, drug therapies were beginning to make rehabilitation possible, and the closing of old purpose-built psychiatric hospitals was on the horizon. Though it was accepted by the 1960s that TCH would be closed in the wake of these changes, no one expected it would take on a new identity as Fairfield Hospital and remain open for another 39 years. In that time it was to adapt to the changes taking place in mental-health thinking and practice.

In the period from the 1970s through to the 1990s there was a distinct move towards community-based care for even those with severe mental-health problems. The 1959 Mental Health Act was instrumental here. Until this radical legislation, many of the long-term in-patients were effectively restricted within the building and only allowed out of it with permission from the consultant or charge nurse. The Act made it abundantly clear that all mental-health patients were voluntary and therefore free to leave unless they were expressly detained in the hospital by one of the defined detention orders newly created by the legislation. These changes reflected the fact that innovative drugs to treat even the most severe psychoses were being developed and they provided, for the first time, at least partial relief from some of the disabling symptoms that affected many of the patients in large hospitals such as Fairfield. Under the 1959 and 1983 Mental Health Acts in-patients were encouraged to work outside the hospital and eventually resettle back into the community with suitable support. Wards such as F3 (within the main hospital) and M10 (a villa ward in the grounds) were set up with a clear remit to rehabilitate patients back into mainstream life. Everyday skills are lost if they are not used regularly and the deficits engendered by institutional living need to be re-learned. Forgotten everyday skills such as budgeting, shopping, using public transport and how to cook were taught in a three-month programme along with social skills and assertiveness training. At the end of this time, working with local housing authorities and support charities, places in the community were identified. Many patients were resettled back with their families while others moved into small flats or, if necessary, into sheltered accommodation. Thus, bit by bit, much of the hospital population was discharged back into society. In the 1990s money was allocated to build wards in the community for those patients whose enduring illness meant they were unable to cope without nursing and medical care.

However, some areas of Fairfield would need to be replaced like-for-like. By the 1980s the Orchard Unit had begun to specialise in low-security forensic care, meaning that some patients were brought in under court orders for offences they had committed while mentally unwell. Before this time it had merely been two locked wards used for the detention of those patients under section who were likely to abscond or who required very intensive nursing care. In its new role as a low-security ward (as against the medium-security specialist units maintained by the government), it would require a replacement unit to be built when Fairfield finally closed its doors. The wards M7 and M8[67] remained one of the most active parts of the hospital, with patients being regularly admitted and discharged even as other wards were closing and the building itself began to be less frequented. The replacement forensic wards were built in the grounds of the Luton & Dunstable Hospital in Luton and called, in memory of its previous incarnation, the Orchard Unit. The transfer of patients across from the now rather dilapidated Fairfield took place in May 1999 and the new unit was officially opened by the Queen in 2000. It was re-named the Robin Pinto Unit in memory of one of its most renowned consultants in 2008.

With the transfer of these last patients the hospital was officially closed in June 1999. Today, the old Three Counties Hospital remains a beautiful and imposing building. Faithfully and sympathetically restored as befits a Grade-II-listed structure, it has been converted into a number of modern apartments. As a testament to the vision of its original architect, George Fowler Jones, the building and grounds remain an impressive 'place in the country'.

Notes

1   LF1/21, Committee of Visitors, Minutes of Visit, 1924

2   Later known as F10. This utilitarian building had no architectural merit and was demolished by the developers in 2001.

3   LF1/23, Dec 1927

4   LF1/23, 136

5   LF1/22, 286

6   Ibid., 132

7   LF1/27, 161

8   LF1/27, 275

9   The first professional educational programme in occupational therapy in the UK (of three years' duration leading to a diploma in occupational therapy) began in 1930 at the Dorset House School of Occupational Therapy in Bristol. The School later relocated to Oxford and eventually the programme was integrated into Oxford Brookes University.

10   http://bedsarchives.bedford.gov.uk/Disability/BromhamHospital.aspx; LF1/29, 56

11   Ex-Fairfield Hospital patient, Alan Suttle, when interviewed in 1998, acknowledged the positive benefits that ECT had on him but also recalled the

fear in which patients held this treatment.

12   Personal conversation between Rory Reynolds and Dr Robert Russell in 1998

13   LF1/29, 253

14   LF1/30

15   LF1/30, 1 Oct 1941

16   LF1/30, 322

17   LF1/32, 12

18   LF1/30, Nov 1940

19   LF1/29, 189

20   LF1/30, 154

21   LF1/31, 124

22   *Ibid.*, 124

23   *Ibid.*, 178

24   LF32, Patient Case Records

25   W. Sargent and E. Slater, *An Introduction to Physical Methods of Treatment in Psychiatry.* Livingstone 1944, 145

26   E. Shorter, *A History of Psychiatry: From the Era of the Asylum to the age of Prozac.* John Wiley & Sons 1997, 227

27   LF1/31, 23 Apr 1945

28   LF1/32, 190

29   LF1/32, 394. The NHS itself was created in 1948 but preparations were well under way immediately after the war.

30   LF1/31, 383

31   LF1/32, 346

32   LF1/32, Nov 1946

33   LF1/32, 186

34   LF1/32, 166, 24 November 1947

35   *Ibid.*, 203

36   From Webster, C. (1988) *The Health Services since the War Vol. 1* (London: HMSO)

37   LF1/32, 297

38   Minutes of Visit, LF2/1, 99

39   The Boards of Control, the successors to the Lunacy Commissioners, were disbanded in 1959

40   In 1960, Monk wrote the first short history of the hospital for the centenary.

41   LF2/1, 322

42   LF4/1/3, Visiting Book, 1952

43   LF2/3, 24 Oct 1957

44   LF2/3, 71

45   LF2/3, 70

46   LF2/3, 169

47   A. Monk, *Fairfield Hospital Centenary, 1860-1960: A Brief History*, privately printed, 1960

48   Reg Buck later became Catering Manager. He retired in 1982

49   Margaret Moor, personal communication.

50   LF2/3, 164

51   LF2/3, 265

52   LF2/3, 271

53   LF2/4, 36

54   The totals in the original document appear to have been incorrectly calculated. We have recalculated them.

55   Hansard: HC Deb 22 July 1954, Vol 530 cc1552–3

56   E. Shorter, 1997, 232

57   LF2/4, 94

58   *Ibid.*, 29 Nov 1954

59   *Ibid.*, 191

60   Letter 14 June 1955. Quoted in Minutes. *Ibid.*, 207

61   LF2/4, 283

62   The title 'Clerk and Steward to the Hospital' was changed in 1948 although it remained in informal use until John Russell's retirement

63   E. Goffman, *Asylums: Essays on the Social Situation of Mental Patients and Other Inmates.* Doubleday 1961, 9

64   HMSO (1962)

65   K. Jones, *Asylums and After: A Revised History of the Mental Health Services from the Early 18th Century to the 1990s.* Athlone Press 1993, 181

66   The banning of patient work was a negative experience for some as Dr Kanakaratnam, consultant psychiatrist, recalled in a 1998 interview: 'When they closed down the farm it was a very sad thing. One particular patient who used to walk around looking very content with himself, afterwards wandered around looking completely lost and he wouldn't engage in any other therapy. There was always an element of industrial therapy at TCH but it was not built up sufficiently to fill the gap. As a result a large number of patients who up to that point had been feeling rather useful suddenly found there was nothing for them.'

67   The terms M7 and M8 denoted two wards in Male wing of the hospital and thus the gender of patients that were kept in them before the 1959 Mental Health Act came into force. After 1970, though, changes were made and it was felt better that the Male and Female locked wards should be as close as possible so the specialist staff could readily move between the wards if there was an emergency. Thus the two wards overlooking the Hospital orchard were selected: Male Ward 8 for the male patients on the upper floor and Male Ward 7 for the females. Within two years, however, it was decided that the wards should be mixed and M8 became the medium security ward and M7, which had access to a large and pleasant walled courtyard , the low security area.

Schedule of Forms of Insanity[1]

I   Congenital or Infantile mental deficiency (Idiocy or Imbecility) occurring as early in life as it can be observed.

Symbols to be entered in the registers
Intellectual –

I 1.*a.*	with Epilepsy
I 1.*b.*	without Epilepsy
I 2.	Moral

II Insanity Occurring Later in Life

Symbols to be entered in the registers

II 1.	Insanity with Epilepsy
II 2.	General Paralysis of the Insane
II 3.	Insanity with the grosser brain lesions
II 4.	Acute delirium (acute delirious mania)
II 5.	Confusional Insanity
II 6.	Stupor
II 7.	Primary Dementia (Dementia Praecox)

Mania –

II 8.*a.*	Recent
II 8.*b.*	Chronic
II 8.*c.*	Recurrent

Melancholia –

II 9.*a.*	Recent
II 9.*b.*	Chronic
II 9.*c.*	Recurrent

II 10.	Alternating Insanity

Delusional Insanity (Paranoia, Paraphrenia)
II 11.*a.* Systematised
II 11.*b.* Non–Systematised

Volitional Insanity –
II 12.*a.* Impulse
II 12.*b.* Obsession
II 12.*c.* Doubt

II 13.   Moral Insanity

Dementia –
II 14.*a.* Senile
II 14.*b.* Secondary or Terminal

Notes

1   Forms 1.B and 2.B of Rules of Commissioners in Lunacy. Case Sheet Index Books, 1912–1932

Index